# Interventional Radiology: Towards Personalized Medicine

# Interventional Radiology: Towards Personalized Medicine

Guest Editor

**Fabio Corvino**

MDPI

Basel • Beijing • Wuhan • Barcelona • Belgrade • Novi Sad • Cluj • Manchester

*Guest Editor*
Fabio Corvino
Azienda Ospedaliera di
Rilievo Nazionale Antonio
Cardarelli
Naples
Italy

*Editorial Office*
MDPI AG
Grosspeteranlage 5
4052 Basel, Switzerland

This is a reprint of the Special Issue, published open access by the journal *Journal of Personalized Medicine* (ISSN 2075-4426), freely accessible at: https://www.mdpi.com/journal/jpm/special_issues/39RR3RZOQL.

For citation purposes, cite each article independently as indicated on the article page online and as indicated below:

| Lastname, A.A.; Lastname, B.B. Article Title. *Journal Name* **Year**, *Volume Number*, Page Range. |
|---|

**ISBN 978-3-7258-6400-3 (Hbk)**
**ISBN 978-3-7258-6401-0 (PDF)**
**https://doi.org/10.3390/books978-3-7258-6401-0**

# Contents

# About the Editor

**Fabio Corvino**

Fabio Corvino, MD, currently works at the Interventional Radiology Unit of AORN Cardarelli Hospital in Naples, Italy. He has been the chief of the junior council of the Italian College of Interventional Radiology (ICIR-SIRM) since 2020. His clinical and research interests include diagnostic and interventional radiology, minimally invasive image-guided procedures, venous and oncologic interventions, and the integration of advanced imaging techniques into personalized therapeutic pathways. He has authored numerous peer-reviewed publications, serves as a reviewer and editorial board member for several international journals, and contributes to national and international research collaborations. His work is dedicated to promoting innovation, education, and evidence-based practice in interventional radiology.

# Preface

The Reprint, "Interventional Radiology towards Personalized Medicine", reflects our intention to provide a clear and unified perspective on how image-guided procedures are reshaping modern clinical practice. The aim of this collection is to present high-quality contributions that demonstrate how technological advancement, refined imaging interpretation, and personalized decision making converge to optimize patient outcomes. The Reprint is addressed to clinicians, radiologists, trainees, and researchers who seek an updated understanding of the expanding potential of interventional radiology across diagnostic and therapeutic pathways. We are grateful to all contributors for their commitment and to the readers who will use these insights to advance patient-centered care.

**Fabio Corvino**
*Guest Editor*

Journal of
*Personalized Medicine*

MDPI

*Editorial*

# Interventional Radiology: Towards Personalized Medicine

**Fabio Corvino** [1,2]

[1] Section of Radiology, Department of Biomedicine, Neuroscience and Advanced Diagnostics (BiND), University Hospital "Paolo Giaccone", 90127 Palermo, Italy; fabio.corvino@unipa.it; Tel.: +39-0817473828
[2] Interventional Radiology Department, AORN "A. Cardarelli", 80131 Naples, Italy

## 1. Introduction

In recent years, the concept of personalized medicine has moved beyond a theoretical framework to become a tangible clinical imperative. The convergence of advanced imaging, minimally invasive therapies, artificial intelligence, and molecular profiling is rapidly transforming conventional care pathways into highly tailored treatment paradigms. Within this evolving landscape, interventional radiology (IR) stands as a core embodiment of precision medicine, uniquely positioned at the intersection of diagnostic insight and real-time therapeutic action. Unlike traditional specialties, which separate diagnostic evaluation from therapeutic intervention, IR unifies both into a single continuum, diagnosing, characterizing, targeting, and treating disease in real time, with millimetric accuracy and minimal invasiveness [1,2].

This Special Issue of the *Journal of Personalized Medicine* was conceived upon the recognition that radiology is no longer a passive observer in the clinical journey. It is an active driver of clinical decision-making, capable of delivering customized solutions that are patient-specific, organ-specific, and even lesion-specific. The contributions gathered in this Special Issue reflect a transformative shift, from generalized therapeutic approaches to tailored interventions guided by imaging biomarkers, functional anatomy, and real-world clinical needs.

Today, IR stands not as an optional adjunct, but as a central pillar of precision medicine, able to individualize treatment, preserve organ function, reduce systemic toxicity, and offer therapeutic options to patients who previously had none. Together, the articles in this Special Issue demonstrate how minimally invasive, image-guided interventions are reshaping oncologic, musculoskeletal, vascular, and trauma care, consolidating IR as a decisive driver of personalized medicine.

## 2. Emerging Themes from the Special Issue: Interventional Radiology as a Catalyst of Personalized Care

The articles featured in this Special Issue collectively demonstrate how IR is expanding the boundaries of personalized medicine across four strategic domains: oncologic precision therapies, organ-preserving trauma management, patient-tailored vascular and pain interventions, and novel imaging-guided procedures for functional restoration. Together, these studies illustrate a paradigm in which treatment is no longer dictated by disease stage alone, but by the individual biological behavior of the lesion, anatomical variability, functional impact, and patient-specific therapeutic goals.

*Precision Oncology: From Image-Guided Diagnosis to Targeted Therapy.* Several contributions underscore the transformative role of interventional oncology, where treatment is guided not only by tumor morphology, but also by functional status, immune environment, and patient physiology (Contribution 1). Holmium-166 radioembolization and sarcopenia monitoring in hepatocellular carcinoma reveal how body composition metrics, derived from imaging, may serve as dynamic biomarkers to predict early tumor progression, paving the way for IR to act as both a therapeutic and prognostic discipline (Contribution 2). Cryoablation of abdominal wall endometriosis and irreversible electroporation for prostate cancer exemplify true personalization: image-guided technologies that adapt the ablation zone based on tissue type, lesion geometry, and patient functional preservation (Contribution 3). Musculoskeletal tumor interventions highlight a tailored oncologic strategy, choosing between ablation, biopsy, or augmentation based on tumor biology and patient prognosis, demonstrating IR's role in curative, palliative, and adjunctive settings (Contribution 4).

*Trauma and Emergency Medicine in the Era of Precision.* Historically managed with uniform surgical strategies, trauma care is being revolutionized by image-guided embolization techniques that allow organ preservation, reduction in surgical morbidity, and individualized hemodynamic management. The multicenter Italian experience in splenic artery embolization shows how the personalized selection of embolization techniques (proximal, distal, or combined) results in consistently high splenic salvage regardless of injury grade, reinforcing IR as the cornerstone of non-operative management (Contribution 5). The review on damage control in liver trauma further illustrates how early endovascular control of bleeding, when integrated within hybrid operating environments, enables tailored interventions for hemodynamically unstable patients, offering time-sensitive, patient-specific solutions (Contribution 6).

*Vascular and Functional Interventions for Personalized Quality-of-Life Care.* Beyond survival, personalized medicine also demands the restoration of function and quality of life. IR is uniquely poised to offer minimally invasive, patient-centric interventions. Prostate artery embolization with small-caliber particles highlights individualized device selection based on vascular anatomy and symptom severity (Contribution 7). Genicular artery embolization for osteoarthritis demonstrates how IR can provide durable pain relief and functional improvement in patients unsuitable for surgery, representing a shift from systemic pharmacotherapy to localized image-guided therapy (Contribution 8).

*Image-Guided Functional Targeting and Anatomical Customization.* The inclusion of innovative techniques, such as ultrasound-guided methylene blue nerve localization, reflects the evolution of IR into a discipline that not only treats structural disease but also modulates function with extreme anatomical precision. This represents the next frontier of personalized medicine: functional intervention tailored to individual anatomy, nerve targeting, and specific motor impairments (Contribution 9).

## 3. Looking Ahead: From Personalized to Predictive and Intelligent Medicine

As medicine transitions from a one-size-fits-all paradigm to a tailored, patient-centered approach, IR is poised not merely to participate in this evolution, but to lead it. The studies presented in this Special Issue collectively demonstrate that precision is no longer defined solely by genetic signatures or pharmacogenomics; it is equally embodied in the ability to visually characterize, selectively target, and therapeutically modify disease in real time. This is the essence of IR, a discipline that does not just align with personalized medicine, but actively enables it.

The next transformative leap will be driven by the integration of artificial intelligence and machine learning into the interventional workflow. Radiomics, AI-based decision support, and predictive modeling will allow interventional radiologists to anticipate treatment response, stratify risk with unprecedented accuracy, and dynamically tailor procedures based on patient-specific anatomy, tumor biology, immune status, and body composition. AI-enhanced imaging interpretation and automated segmentation are transforming the interventional suite into a data-driven, intelligent environment, one in which diagnosis and therapy are no longer sequential phases but part of a continuous, adaptive process [3,4].

In this framework, IR becomes the operational engine of precision medicine, transforming imaging from a diagnostic endpoint into a therapeutic roadmap powered by real-time analytics and AI-derived biomarkers. The future of patient care will be image-guided, minimally invasive, data-enriched, and continuously optimized, where every intervention is not only targeted, but *intelligently* tailored to the unique biological and functional profile of each patient [5].

Rather than marking an endpoint, this Special Issue inaugurates a new era in which image-guided therapies, empowered by artificial intelligence, redefine standards of care, improve quality of life, and bridge the gap between diagnosis, prediction, and cure. IR, increasingly supported by data-driven decision tools, stands ready to drive the next great transformation in modern medicine.

**Conflicts of Interest:** The author declare no conflicts of interest.

**List of Contributions:**

1. Faiella, E.; Santucci, D.; Vertulli, D.; Vergantino, E.; Vaccarino, F.; Perillo, G.; Beomonte Zobel, B.; Grasso, R.F. Irreversible Electroporation (IRE) for Prostate Cancer (PCa) Treatment: The State of the Art. *J. Pers. Med.* **2024**, *14*, 137. https://doi.org/10.3390/jpm14020137.
2. Trobiani, C.; Ubaldi, N.; Teodoli, L.; Tipaldi, M.A.; Cappelli, F.; Ungania, S.; Vallati, G. The Deterioration of Sarcopenia Post-Transarterial Radioembolization with Holmium-166 Serves as a Predictor for Disease Progression at 3 Months in Patients with Advanced Hepatocellular Carcinoma: A Pilot Study. *J. Pers. Med.* **2024**, *14*, 511. https://doi.org/10.3390/jpm14050511.
3. Touimi Benjelloun, G.; Mokbli, M.; Kammoun, T.; Ghabri, S.; Sammoud, S.; Nabi, W.; Letouzey, V.; Beregi, J.-P.; Frandon, J. Efficacy and Safety of Personalized Percutaneous Single-Probe Cryoablation Using Liquid Nitrogen in the Treatment of Abdominal Wall Endometriosis. *J. Pers. Med.* **2025**, *15*, 373. https://doi.org/10.3390/jpm15080373.
4. Uldin, H.; Kanbour, I.; Patel, A.; Botchu, R. Image-Guided Musculoskeletal Interventional Radiology in the Personalised Management of Musculoskeletal Tumours. *J. Pers. Med.* **2024**, *14*, 1167. https://doi.org/10.3390/jpm14121167.
5. Corvino, F.; Giurazza, F.; Tipaldi, M.A.; Rossi, T.; Daviddi, F.; Perrone, O.; Ambrosini, I.; D'addato, M.; Villanova, I.; Marra, P.; et al. Real-World Outcomes of Splenic Artery Embolization in Blunt Splenic Trauma: Insights from an Italian Multicenter Cohort. *J. Pers. Med.* **2025**, *15*, 420. https://doi.org/10.3390/jpm15090420.
6. Corvino, F.; Giurazza, F.; Marra, P.; Ierardi, A.M.; Corvino, A.; Basile, A.; Galia, M.; Inzerillo, A.; Niola, R. Damage Control Interventional Radiology in Liver Trauma: A Comprehensive Review. *J. Pers. Med.* **2024**, *14*, 365. https://doi.org/10.3390/jpm14040365.
7. Xhepa, G.; Sciacqua, L.V.; Vanzulli, A.; Canì, A.E.; Ascenti, V.; Ricoeur, A.; Ianniello, A.A.; Inzerillo, A.; Nicotera, P.; Del Grande, F.; et al. Prostate Artery Embolization (PAE) with Small Beads for the Treatment of Benign Prostatic Hyperplasia (BPH). *J. Pers. Med.* **2024**, *14*, 613. https://doi.org/10.3390/jpm14060613.
8. Femia, M.; Valenti Pittino, C.; Fumarola, E.M.; Tramarin, M.; Papa, M.; Giurazza, F.; Francioso, A.P.; Fior, D.; Moramarco, L.P.; Antonini, G.; et al. Genicular Artery Embolization: A New Tool for the Management of Refractory Osteoarthritis-Related Knee Pain. *J. Pers. Med.* **2024**, *14*, 686. https://doi.org/10.3390/jpm14070686.
9. Zerbinati, P.; Bemporad, J.; Massimiani, A.; Bianchini, E.; Mazzoli, D.; Glorioso, D.; della Vecchia, G.; De Luca, A.; De Blasiis, P. Lateral Pectoral Nerve Identification through Ultrasound-Guided Methylene Blue Injection during Selective Peripheral Neurectomy for Shoulder Spasticity: Proposal for a New Procedure. *J. Pers. Med.* **2024**, *14*, 116. https://doi.org/10.3390/jpm14010116.

## References

1. Ji, J.; Fang, S.; Chen, M.; Zheng, L.; Chen, W.; Zhao, Z.; Cheng, Y. Precision interventional radiology. *J. Interv. Med.* **2021**, *4*, 155–158. [CrossRef] [PubMed] [PubMed Central]
2. Brock, K.K.; Chen, S.R.; Sheth, R.A.; Siewerdsen, J.H. Imaging in Interventional Radiology: 2043 and Beyond. *Radiology* **2023**, *308*, e230146. [CrossRef] [PubMed] [PubMed Central]
3. Seah, J.; Boeken, T.; Sapoval, M.; Goh, G.S. Prime Time for Artificial Intelligence in Interventional Radiology. *Cardiovasc. Interv. Radiol.* **2022**, *45*, 283–289. [CrossRef] [PubMed] [PubMed Central]
4. Handelman, G.S.; Kok, H.K.; Chandra, R.V.; Razavi, A.H.; Lee, M.J.; Asadi, H. eDoctor: Machine learning and the future of medicine. *J. Intern. Med.* **2018**, *284*, 603–619. [CrossRef] [PubMed]
5. Najafi, G.; Kreiser, K.; Abdelaziz, M.E.M.K.; Hamady, M.S. Current State of Robotics in Interventional Radiology. *Cardiovasc. Interv. Radiol.* **2023**, *46*, 549–561. [CrossRef] [PubMed] [PubMed Central]

Journal of
*Personalized Medicine*

MDPI

*Article*

# Real-World Outcomes of Splenic Artery Embolization in Blunt Splenic Trauma: Insights from an Italian Multicenter Cohort

**Fabio Corvino [1,*], Francesco Giurazza [1], Marcello Andrea Tipaldi [2], Tommaso Rossi [3], Francesco Daviddi [4], Orsola Perrone [4], Ilaria Ambrosini [4], Mauro D'addato [5], Ilaria Villanova [5], Paolo Marra [6,7], Francesco Saverio Carbone [6], Antonio Vizzuso [8], Fernando Smaldone [8], Anna Rita Scrofani [9], Roberto Iezzi [9], Andrea Discalzi [10], Marco Calandri [11], Marco Femia [12], Carlo Valenti Pittino [12], Ruggero Vercelli [12], Daniele Falsaperla [13], Antonello Basile [13], Antonio Bruno [14], Chiara Gasperini [14] and Raffaella Niola [1]**

1 Interventional Radiology Department, AORN "A. Cardarelli", 80131 Naples, Italy; francesco.giurazza@aocardarelli.it (F.G.)
2 Department of Surgical and Medical Sciences and Translational Medicine, Sapienza-University of Rome, 00189 Rome, Italy
3 Department of Radiological Sciences, Oncology and Pathology, Policlinico Umberto I Hospital, Sapienza University of Rome, Viale del Policlinico 155 Sapienza, 00161 Rome, Italy
4 UO Radiologia Interventistica, Azienda Ospedaliera Universitaria Pisa A.O.U.P., 56126 Pisa, Italy
5 Azienda Ospedaliero-Consorziale Policlinico di Bari, P.za Giulio Cesare, 70124 Bari, Italy
6 Department of Radiology, AAST Papa Giovanni XXIII Hospital, 24127 Bergamo, Italy
7 School of Medicine and Surgery, University of Milano-Bicocca, 20126 Milano, Italy
8 Radiology Unit, Morgagni-Pierantoni Hospital, AUSL Romagna, 47121 Forlì, Italy
9 Department of Diagnostic Imaging, Oncologic Radiotherapy and Hematology, Fondazione Policlinico Universitario Agostino Gemelli IRCCS, 00168 Rome, Italy
10 Department of Diagnostic Imaging and Interventional Radiology, City of Health and Science University Hospital, University of Turin, 10126 Turin, Italy
11 Department of Surgical Sciences, University of Turin, 10126 Turin, Italy
12 Interventional Radiology Unit, ASST Santi Paolo Carlo, 20122 Milan, Italy
13 Department of Medical Surgical Sciences and Advanced Technologies "GF Ingrassia", University Hospital Policlinico "G. Rodolico-San Marco", 95123 Catania, Italy
14 Diagnostic and Interventional Radiology Unit, Maggiore Hospital "C. A. Pizzardi", 40133 Bologna, Italy
* Correspondence: fabio.corvino@aocardarelli.it; Tel.: +39-3334530499 or +39-0817473828

**Abstract: Background:** Splenic artery embolization (SAE) has emerged as a key adjunct to non-operative management (NOM) in hemodynamically stable patients with blunt splenic trauma, yet variability in its application persists across centers. **Objectives:** The aim was to evaluate real-life clinical practices, techniques, and outcomes of SAE in blunt splenic trauma across multiple Italian trauma centers. **Materials and Methods:** This retrospective multicenter study analyzed data from 281 patients undergoing emergency SAE for blunt splenic trauma between January 2019 and December 2021. Demographics, imaging findings, embolization techniques, complications, and outcomes were collected and analyzed. Multivariate logistic regression was used to assess predictors of splenectomy. **Results:** The technical success rate was 100%, with a 9.6% rate of post-embolization splenectomy and a complication rate of 24.9% (including 5.7% splenic infarction and 3.2% rebleeding). Embolization was performed proximally (46.6%), distally (28.8%), or with a combined approach (24.6%). No significant correlation was found between embolization technique and splenectomy rate. Patients with AAST grade III injuries benefited from SAE with high technical success and low failure rates. Notably, 14.2% of patients underwent angiography despite negative CT, with a splenectomy rate of 10% in this subgroup. Multivariate analysis identified no independent predictors of splenectomy. **Conclusions:** SAE is a reliable and effective tool in the management of blunt splenic trauma, achieving high splenic salvage rates even in selected grade III injuries and CT-negative patients. In an era of precision medicine, interventional radiology should be regarded as a distinct and specific treatment modality, comparable to surgery, rather than being merely included within non-operative management (NOM).

**Keywords:** splenic trauma; splenic artery embolization; non-operative management; interventional radiology; AAST grading; splenic salvage; trauma management

## 1. Introduction

Splenic trauma is one of the most common intra-abdominal injuries encountered in blunt trauma cases, with the spleen being the most frequently affected solid organ. Over the past decades, the management of splenic trauma has significantly evolved, shifting from an exclusively surgical approach to a predominantly non-operative management (NOM) strategy. This transition has been driven primarily by a deeper understanding of the spleen's immunological functions and the associated risks of splenectomy, notably overwhelming post-splenectomy infections (OPSIs). Consequently, splenic artery embolization (SAE) has become a crucial adjunctive procedure in NOM, enhancing the preservation of the spleen in hemodynamically stable patients, particularly those with high-grade injuries [1,2].

According to the latest guidelines from the World Society of Emergency Surgery (WSES), SAE is recommended in patients with AAST grade III–V splenic injuries who are hemodynamically stable or transient responders [3]. Previous studies have consistently demonstrated that SAE significantly reduces the need for surgical intervention while maintaining high rates of splenic salvage. Despite widespread adoption, considerable variability persists in clinical practice, particularly regarding embolization techniques [4,5]. Distal SAE is usually indicated for focal vascular injuries, such as pseudoaneurysms and active extravasation, whereas proximal SAE aims primarily to reduce arterial pressure and facilitate hemostasis without inducing extensive infarction, relying on collateral circulation to maintain splenic viability. Nonetheless, there remains an ongoing debate as to whether proximal embolization should be routinely performed in AAST grade IV injuries or selectively applied in grade III cases [6–8].

In Italy, clinical practice regarding SAE in splenic trauma appears to be heterogeneous, and assessing a realistic national splenectomy rate is currently challenging due to the lack of readily accessible and centralized data, which stems from the absence of a national trauma registry dedicated to interventional procedures. Therefore, evaluating real-life outcomes and identifying common practice patterns through multicenter Italian data is essential. This multicenter, retrospective observational study aims to provide a comprehensive analysis of SAE across several major Italian trauma centers, specifically assessing embolization techniques, clinical outcomes, and factors influencing the rate of splenectomy. By presenting real-world evidence from diverse Italian centers, this study seeks to establish a baseline understanding of current clinical practice, highlight critical trends, and contribute valuable data for future standardization efforts and optimization of SAE protocols at a national level.

## 2. Materials and Methods

### *2.1. Patient Selection and Data Collection*

All patients who underwent emergency SAE following blunt abdominal trauma between January 2019 and December 2021 were included in this study. This study focused on patients who underwent SAE for blunt splenic trauma; individuals managed with primary splenectomy or other non-interventional approaches were not included, as they were outside the scope of the analysis. The cohort was composed of consecutive patients from 11

Italian trauma centers, identified in the Author Affiliations Section. Table 1 summarizes the distribution of patients and key demographic characteristics across the participating centers. Each center contributed retrospectively collected cases managed with emergency SAE between January 2019 and December 2021, using a standardized data collection protocol. The study period (January 2019–December 2021) was chosen to ensure a uniform retrospective data window across participating centers, allowing complete in-hospital outcome assessment. All submitted data were centrally curated at the coordinating center (A.O.R.N. A. Cardarelli, Naples). Manual verification was performed to identify and correct inconsistencies, missing values, or outliers through direct communication with participating centers prior to analysis. The data collection period spanned from January 2019 to December 2021. Data curation and quality control were performed between early 2022 and mid-2023, followed by statistical analysis and manuscript drafting. The final submission of the study occurred in 2025. Data collected included patient age, sex, trauma date, angiography date, and time elapsed between trauma and embolization. A standardized Excel-based data collection form was distributed to each participating center to ensure uniformity (Supplementary Table S1). Centralized curation of data was performed, including manual verification of outliers and correction of any missing or implausible values prior to analysis.

**Table 1.** Distribution of patients and demographic characteristics across the 11 participating centers. The order of centers does not reflect relative importance but follows the order of appearance of author affiliations in the manuscript.

| Institution | N. Patients | Mean Age ± SD (Years) | Male | Female |
|---|---|---|---|---|
| Interventional Radiology Department—AORN "A. Cardarelli", Naples | 49 | 46 ± 20 | 36 | 12 |
| Interventional Radiology Unit—Sant'Andrea Hospital of Rome, Rome | 8 | 59 ± 22 | 3 | 5 |
| UO Interventional Radiology—A.O.U.P., Pisa | 26 | 47 ± 20 | 18 | 8 |
| Radiology Unit—A.O.C. Policlinico di Bari, Bari | 9 | 57 ± 15 | 8 | 1 |
| Department of Radiology—AAST Papa Giovanni XXIII, Bergamo | 24 | 43 ± 24 | 19 | 5 |
| Radiology Unit, Morgagni-Pierantoni Hospital—AUSL Romagna, Forlì | 48 | 51 ± 21 | 21 | 26 |
| Department of Diagnostic Imaging, Oncologic Radiotherapy and Hematology—"Fondazione Policlinico Universitario Agostino Gemelli IRCCS", Roma | 17 | 56 ± 21 | 12 | 5 |
| Department of Diagnostic Imaging and Interventional Radiology—City of Health and Science University Hospital—University of Turin, Turin | 36 | 43 ± 19 | 27 | 9 |
| Interventional Radiology Unit—ASST Santi Paolo Carlo, Milano | 9 | 49 ± 27 | 6 | 3 |
| Radiology Unit 1—University Hospital Policlinico "G. Rodolico-San Marco", Catania | 7 | 49 ± 22 | 4 | 1 |
| Diagnostic and Interventional Radiology Unit—Maggiore Hospital "C. A. Pizzardi", Bologna | 48 | 46 ± 20 | 36 | 12 |

*2.2. Radiological and Procedural Parameters*

All patients underwent contrast-enhanced computed tomography (CT) prior to digital subtraction angiography (DSA). The presence of vascular injuries, such as active contrast extravasation or pseudoaneurysm, was classified as either present or absent. Splenic injury severity was assessed according to the 2018 AAST grading system. Hemoperitoneum was categorized as grade I (localized, e.g., perisplenic, perihepatic, Morrison's pouch), grade II (extension to paracolic gutters), or grade III (pelvic involvement). SAE was classified according to the embolization site as proximal, distal, or combined. Embolic materials were documented and included pushable or detachable coils (0.035″ or 0.018″), vascular plugs, gelatin sponge (Spongostan), glue, and polyvinyl alcohol (PVA) particles. However, data concerning embolic materials were highly heterogeneous, reflecting significant variability among centers due to differing local expertise. Therefore, an accurate and detailed evaluation of embolic materials was not feasible in this analysis. Due to this heterogeneity and lack of standardized protocols, embolic materials were excluded from comparative outcome analysis.

### 2.3. Outcome Definitions

Technical success was defined as the absence of vascular lesions or active bleeding at the post-embolization angiographic control. Complications were classified according to the Cardiovascular and Interventional Radiological Society of Europe (CIRSE) guidelines and included splenic infarction, rebleeding, splenectomy, and non-target embolization [9]. Splenectomy was defined as any surgical removal of the spleen following embolization, with the time from embolization to surgery recorded in hours.

### 2.4. Statistical Analysis

Descriptive statistics, including the mean, standard deviation (SD), median, interquartile range (IQR), and proportions, were calculated for all demographic, clinical, radiological, and procedural variables. Relationships between embolization techniques and clinical outcomes were evaluated using Chi-square or Fisher's exact tests for categorical variables and Mann–Whitney U tests for non-parametric continuous data, due to the non-normal distribution and small group sizes in several cases.

Logistic regression analysis was performed to identify potential predictors of splenectomy, which represented the main clinical outcome of interest. Independent variables were selected based on clinical relevance and preliminary univariate analyses and included AAST grade, embolization type, presence of vascular injury at CT and DSA, and time from trauma to embolization. Multivariate logistic regression was performed using a complete-case analysis approach: patients with missing values for any of the variables included in the model were excluded from this part of the analysis.

Given the limited number of splenectomy events, a sensitivity analysis was additionally performed using Firth's penalized logistic regression to account for potential small-sample bias and sparse data structure. This approach improves the reliability of estimates in the context of low event rates. The results of this penalized model are presented in Supplementary Table S2.

All statistical analyses were performed using Python 3.9.7 (libraries: Pandas, SciPy, Statsmodels). A $p$-value < 0.05 was considered statistically significant.

## 3. Results

### 3.1. Patient Population

A total of 281 patients from 11 Italian centers were analyzed. The mean age was 41.3 ± 17.8 years, with a predominance of males (75.4%). The median time from trauma to embolization was 8.5 h (IQR 4.0–17.8), indicating timely management in most cases. In a minority of cases ($n$ = 2), embolization was performed more than 72 h after trauma due to delayed complications such as secondary bleeding. These cases were retained in the analysis as they represent real-life clinical scenarios. A comprehensive summary of the demographic and clinical variables is provided in Table 2.

**Table 2.** Cumulative summary table of study population.

| Parameter | Value |
|---|---|
| Total number of patients | 281 |
| Mean age ± SD (years) | 41.3 ± 17.8 |
| Male/Female | 191/90 |
| Mean time trauma to embolization (h) ± SD | 35.7 ± 80.4 |
| Range of time trauma to embolization (h) | 0.5–600.0 |
| AAST grade distribution (III-V) | 2: 30 (10.7%);<br>3: 61 (21.7%);<br>4: 176 (62.6%);<br>5: 14 (5.0%) |
| Embolization type distribution<br>P = proximal embolization; D = distal embolization; C = combined proximal and distal embolization | P: 161 (57.3%);<br>D: 84 (29.9%);<br>C: 36 (12.8%) |
| Number of complications | 70 (24.9%) |
| Number of splenectomies | 27 (9.6%) |

### 3.2. Injury Severity and Imaging Findings

According to the 2018 AAST classification, injury distribution was as follows: grades I–II: 13 (4.6%); grade III: 53 patients (18.9%); grade IV: 149 (53.0%); grade V: 66 (23.5%). Baseline CT identified vascular injuries in 217 (77.2%) cases, whereas angiography confirmed vascular injuries in 256 patients (91.1%). Forty patients (14.2%) underwent embolization despite negative CT findings but had positive DSA results, predominantly among low-grade injuries (AAST I–III). These findings support the role of DSA as a complementary diagnostic tool in cases where CT findings are inconclusive, especially in hemodynamically stable patients with ongoing clinical suspicion.

### 3.3. Embolization Technique and Procedural Details

SAE was categorized as proximal (131 patients, 46.6%), distal (81 patients, 28.8%), and combined proximal–distal (69 patients, 24.6%). The technical success rate was 100%, defined as complete vascular lesion exclusion at post-embolization DSA. Table 3 summarizes the complication distribution and splenectomy rates.

**Table 3.** Distribution of complications and splenectomy rates according to embolization technique.

| Embolization Type | Total Patients | Splenic Infarction | Rebleeding | Non-Target Embolization | Splenectomy |
|---|---|---|---|---|---|
| Combined | 36 | 2 | 2 | 2 | 1 |
| Distal | 84 | 8 | 9 | 0 | 10 |
| Proximal | 161 | 10 | 4 | 21 | 16 |

### 3.4. Post-Procedural Outcomes and Complications

A total of 70 patients (24.9%) experienced complications according to CIRSE classification. These included splenic infarction (16 cases, 5.7%), rebleeding (9 cases, 3.2%), and non-target embolization (2 cases, 0.7%). Additionally, splenectomy was performed in 27 patients (9.6%) due to clinical deterioration. However, splenectomy in this context is not regarded as a procedural complication but rather as a failure of NOM, despite technically successful embolization. No statistically significant association was found between embolization technique and splenectomy rate ($p = 0.526$) or between AAST grade and splenectomy ($p = 0.713$), although grade V injuries trended toward higher splenectomy rates.

### 3.5. Multivariate Analysis

Multivariate logistic regression analysis did not identify any statistically significant independent predictors of splenectomy among the evaluated variables (AAST grade, embolization type, presence of vascular injury at CT and angiography, and time from trauma to embolization). However, patients with higher-grade splenic injuries (AAST IV–V) showed a non-significant trend toward increased odds of requiring splenectomy compared to those with lower-grade injuries (AAST I–III) (odds ratio [OR] 2.11, 95% confidence interval [CI] 0.93–4.38, $p = 0.074$). No relevant trends were observed for embolization technique or timing. These findings are visually summarized in the forest plot presented in Figure 1, which illustrates the odds ratios and confidence intervals for all variables included in the regression model.

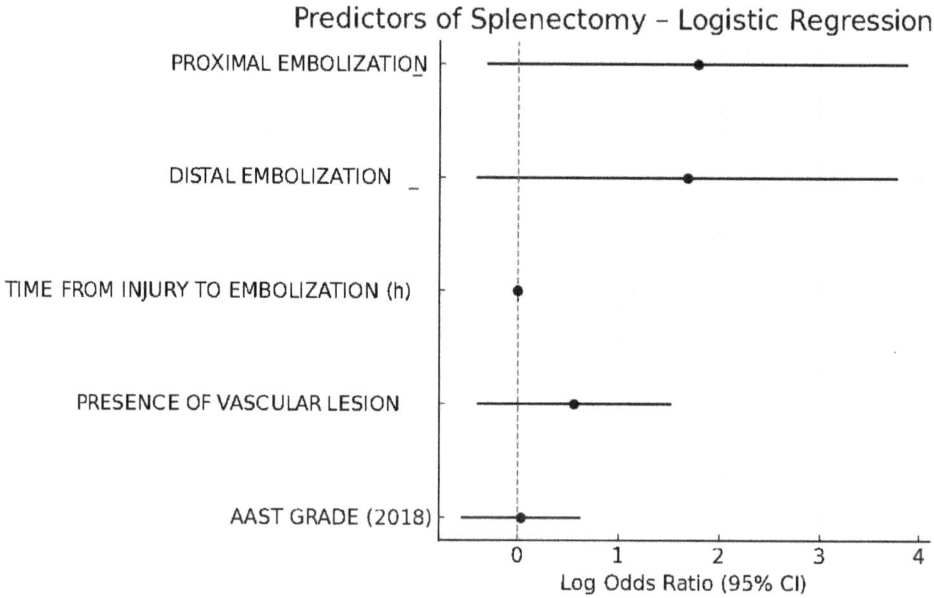


**Figure 1.** Forest plot of logistic regression analysis showing independent predictors of splenectomy after embolization in patients with blunt splenic trauma. The plot reports the OR and 95% CI for each variable. Although proximal and distal embolization showed higher odds ratios in the regression model, none of the variables—including embolization technique, AAST grade, time to embolization, and presence of vascular lesion—reached statistical significance as independent predictors of splenectomy. The dashed vertical line indicates the null value (OR = 1).

### 3.6. Subgroup Analysis

Of 40 patients with negative CT but positive angiographic findings, 34 (85%) had AAST grade II–III injuries, while 6 (15%) had high-grade (AAST IV) lesions. These patients underwent angiography despite the absence of CT-evident vascular injury due to persistent clinical suspicion, such as unexplained hemodynamic instability, hemoglobin drop, or equivocal imaging findings. Four patients (10%) ultimately required splenectomy. The embolization rate in this subgroup was comparable to that of CT-positive patients. The AAST grade distribution within this subgroup is shown in Figure 2, highlighting the diagnostic and therapeutic value of angiography in selected trauma cases with inconclusive CT results.

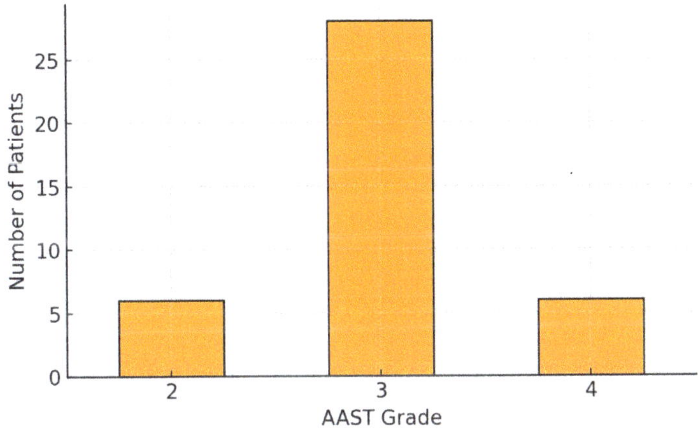


**Figure 2.** Distribution of AAST grades in the subgroup of patients with negative CT findings but positive angiographic evidence of vascular injury ($n$ = 40). The majority of patients had intermediate-grade injuries (AAST III, 70%), while low-grade (AAST II) and high-grade (AAST IV) lesions were less common, each accounting for 15% of the subgroup.

## 4. Discussion

This large multicenter study offers one of the most extensive real-life evaluations of SAE in Italy to date, providing a robust overview of current interventional strategies for blunt splenic trauma. The findings confirm the widespread adoption of SAE as an effective adjunct to NOM in blunt splenic trauma, particularly for hemodynamically stable patients with moderate-to-severe injuries (AAST grades III–V).

Our results highlight a 100% technical success rate and a relatively low rate of splenectomy (9.6%), in line with previously published data. However, the overall complication rate (24.9%)—including infarction, rebleeding, and splenectomy—emphasizes that SAE, while minimally invasive, is not without risks. As noted in Rasuli et al., complications may be underreported in some series, particularly infarction, which varies in incidence depending on the embolization technique and extent [10].

The high frequency of splenic infarction observed after distal embolization should not be interpreted as a traditional complication. The spleen's terminal vascularization, particularly at the segmental and subsegmental levels, makes focal infarction a predictable outcome when performing superselective embolization. These areas are usually self-limited and clinically silent, rarely requiring treatment [11,12].

Furthermore, several studies have shown that distal embolization, despite causing partial infarction, is associated with preservation of overall splenic immune function. As demonstrated by Foley et al., patients treated with both proximal and distal embolization had significantly higher levels of circulating IgM memory B cells compared to splenectomized patients, with a trend toward better immunologic preservation in the distal embolization group [8–13]. This observation reinforces the concept that infarction of limited parenchymal areas does not compromise the spleen's immunological role and should not be regarded as an adverse outcome.

In our study, splenectomy was not classified as a procedural complication of splenic artery embolization, but rather as an outcome indicating failure of NOM, consistent with the classification proposed in the WSES guidelines. According to these recommendations, splenectomy following SAE is typically related to persistent or recurrent bleeding rather than technical failure of the embolization procedure itself. This distinction is important to accurately interpret SAE outcomes in real-world trauma settings [14].

A notable aspect of our study was the inclusion of a subgroup of 40 patients who underwent angiography despite the absence of vascular injury on CT. Among these, 85% had intermediate-grade (AAST I–III) injuries, and yet 10% eventually required splenectomy. This subgroup exemplifies a real-life clinical dilemma: persistent clinical signs (tachycardia, hypotension, falling hemoglobin level) may prompt angiography even in the absence of radiological evidence. This practice is supported by Yoo et al., who showed that embolization in CT-negative but high-suspicion trauma patients may improve splenic salvage. Thus, our findings advocate for a selective use of angiography in patients with incongruent clinical and radiological profiles, especially when institutional expertise permits [15].

Another unresolved issue remains the indication for SAE in AAST grade III injuries. While WSES guidelines endorse SAE for grades III–V, many studies still limit embolization to higher grades or clear evidence of vascular injury. Our study included 53 patients with grade III injuries, of whom a substantial number underwent embolization—either due to CT-positive vascular findings or clinical suspicion. Notably, this subgroup achieved high technical success and low splenectomy rates, suggesting that SAE may be a valid therapeutic option even in selected grade III injuries. However, this remains controversial: some authors, like Gasparetto et al. argue that embolization in AAST III should be reserved for cases with contrast blush or pseudoaneurysm, while others, such as Tidadini F et al., support a more liberal approach to prevent delayed bleeding [16,17]. This variability underscores the need for individualized decision-making based on hemodynamic status, imaging, and institutional experience.

Moreover, multivariate analysis in our cohort did not identify statistically significant predictors of splenectomy. Nevertheless, a trend toward increased odds of splenectomy in higher AAST grades was observed, aligning with findings from the literature [18,19]. Embolization type did not influence outcomes, suggesting that technique selection may reflect anatomical and operator factors rather than efficacy [1,20].

Our results are in line with those reported by Gill et al. [21], who confirmed the safety and efficacy of SAE in a Level 1 trauma center setting, with similar splenic salvage rates and complication profiles. Likewise, Lin et al. [22] provided further evidence on the equivalence of proximal, distal, and combined embolization approaches in terms of clinical outcomes, supporting the flexibility of SAE technique selection in real-world trauma care.

The limitations of this study include its retrospective design, heterogeneity in embolization technique and material across centers, and lack of long-term follow-up regarding immunological outcomes or late complications. However, the large sample size, multicenter nature, and inclusion of real-life data provide a valuable contribution to the ongoing debate on optimal SAE strategies in blunt splenic trauma.

In conclusion, our experience demonstrates that splenic artery embolization—particularly when tailored according to vascular injury patterns—is a reliable and effective strategy in the non-operative management of blunt splenic trauma. Its clinical efficacy and safety profile render it comparable to surgical treatment in selected cases, especially in high-grade injuries (AAST grade III and above), which traditionally posed significant management challenges. In light of these results, future guidelines should adopt a three-tiered approach to splenic trauma treatment: (1) NOM, (2) interventional radiological treatment, (3) surgical intervention. In an era of precision medicine, recognizing interventional radiology (IR) as a distinct and primary therapeutic option is crucial to optimize outcomes, reduce unnecessary splenectomies, and preserve organ function in trauma patients. This perspective is increasingly reflected in current trauma management frameworks. The latest WSES guidelines explicitly recommend SAE as a first-line treatment in hemodynamically stable patients with high-grade splenic injuries (AAST III–V) or signs of vascular injury. Similarly, the Eastern Association for the Surgery of Trauma (EAST) and Advanced Trauma

Life Support (ATLS) guidelines incorporate embolization into the standard algorithm for blunt splenic trauma [3,23,24]. These positions support the view that IR should be regarded as an autonomous pillar—alongside conservative and surgical approaches—within a modern, tiered treatment strategy for splenic trauma.

**Supplementary Materials:** The following supporting information can be downloaded at: https://www.mdpi.com/article/10.3390/jpm15090420/s1, Table S1: Data collection grid; Table S2: Results of Firth's penalized logistic regression.

**Author Contributions:** Conceptualization, F.C. and M.A.T.; methodology, F.G., T.R. and R.N.; software, F.D., I.A. and O.P.; validation, M.D., I.V. and P.M.; formal analysis, F.S.C. and A.V.; investigation, A.R.S., F.S. and R.I.; resources, F.C. and C.G.; data curation, F.C., A.D., M.C. and M.F.; writing—original draft preparation, F.C.; writing—review and editing, C.V.P., A.B. (Antonello Basile) and R.N.; visualization, R.V., D.F. and A.B. (Antonio Bruno); supervision, F.C. and R.N. All authors have read and agreed to the published version of the manuscript.

**Funding:** This research received no external funding.

**Institutional Review Board Statement:** This study was conducted in accordance with the ethical principles of the Declaration of Helsinki. Ethical review and approval were waived in accordance with national and European regulations (EU Regulation 2016/679—GDPR and Italian Legislative Decree 101/2018), as this was a non-interventional, retrospective analysis of anonymized data collected during routine clinical practice. No identifiable personal data were processed, and all analyses were conducted in aggregate form, exempting the study from formal Ethics Committee approval.

**Informed Consent Statement:** Informed consent was obtained from all subjects involved in this study.

**Data Availability Statement:** The data presented in this study are not publicly available due to privacy and ethical restrictions, as they contain sensitive clinical information from multiple institutions and were not collected with prior consent for public sharing.

**Conflicts of Interest:** The authors declare no conflicts of interest.

## References

1. Habash, M.; Ceballos, D.; Gunn, A.J. Splenic Artery Embolization for Patients with High-Grade Splenic Trauma: Indications, Techniques, and Clinical Outcomes. *Semin. Intervent Radiol.* **2021**, *38*, 105–112. [CrossRef] [PubMed] [PubMed Central]
2. Schnüriger, B.; Inaba, K.; Konstantinidis, A.; Lustenberger, T.; Chan, L.S.; Demetriades, D. Outcomes of proximal versus distal splenic artery embolization after trauma: A systematic review and meta-analysis. *J. Trauma: Inj. Infect. Crit. Care* **2011**, *70*, 252–260. [CrossRef] [PubMed]
3. Coccolini, F.; Montori, G.; Catena, F.; Kluger, Y.; Biffl, W.; Moore, E.E.; Reva, V.; Bing, C.; Bala, M.; Fugazzola, P.; et al. Splenic trauma: WSES classification and guidelines for adult and pediatric patients. *World J. Emerg. Surg.* **2017**, *12*, 40. [CrossRef] [PubMed] [PubMed Central]
4. Clements, W.; Woolley, I.; Zia, A.; Kavnoudias, H.; Weber, D.G.; Spelman, D.W.; Mathew, J. A nationwide Australian cross-sectional study assessing current management and infection prevention practices after Splenic Artery Embolisation (SAE) following trauma. *Injury* **2025**, *56*, 112593. [CrossRef] [PubMed]
5. Clements, W.; Joseph, T.; Koukounaras, J.; Goh, G.S.; Moriarty, H.K.; Mathew, J.; Phan, T.D. SPLEnic salvage and complications after splenic artery EmbolizatioN for blunt abdomINal trauma: The SPLEEN-IN study. *CVIR Endovasc.* **2020**, *3*, 92. [CrossRef] [PubMed] [PubMed Central]
6. Corvino, F.; Giurazza, F.; Ierardi, A.M.; Lucatelli, P.; Basile, A.; Corvino, A.; Niola, R. Splenic Artery Pseudoaneurysms: The Role of ce-CT for Diagnosis and Treatment Planning. *Diagnostics* **2022**, *12*, 1012. [CrossRef] [PubMed] [PubMed Central]
7. Quencer, K.B.; Smith, T.A. Review of proximal splenic artery embolization in blunt abdominal trauma. *CVIR Endovasc.* **2019**, *2*, 11. [CrossRef] [PubMed] [PubMed Central]
8. Foley, P.T.; Kavnoudias, H.; Cameron, P.U.; Czarnecki, C.; Paul, E.; Lyon, S.M. Proximal Versus Distal Splenic Artery Embolisation for Blunt Splenic Trauma: What is the Impact on Splenic Immune Function? *Cardiovasc. Intervent Radiol.* **2015**, *38*, 1143–1151. [CrossRef] [PubMed]

9. Filippiadis, D.K.; Binkert, C.; Pellerin, O.; Hoffmann, R.T.; Krajina, A.; Pereira, P.L. Cirse Quality Assurance Document and Standards for Classification of Complications: The Cirse Classification System. *Cardiovasc. Intervent Radiol.* **2017**, *40*, 1141–1146. [CrossRef] [PubMed]
10. Rasuli, P.; Moosavi, B.; French, G.J.; Petrcich, W.; Hammond, I. Splenic Artery Embolization in Blunt Trauma: A Single-Center Retrospective Comparison of the Use of Gelatin Sponge Versus Coils. *Am. J. Roentgenol.* **2017**, *209*, W382–W387. [CrossRef]
11. Talwar, A.; Knight, G.; Al Asadi, A.; Entezari, P.; Chen, R.; Resnick, S.; Komanduri, S.; Gabr, A.; Thornburg, B.; Salem, R.; et al. Post-embolization outcomes of splenic artery pseudoaneurysms: A single-center experience. *Clin. Imaging* **2021**, *80*, 160–166. [CrossRef] [PubMed]
12. Entriken, C.; Weed, Z.; Parikh, P.P.; Ekeh, A.P. Complications Following Splenic Embolization for Trauma: Have Things Changed Over Time? *J. Surg. Res.* **2022**, *277*, 44–49. [CrossRef] [PubMed]
13. Slater, S.J.; Lukies, M.; Kavnoudias, H.; Zia, A.; Lee, R.; Bosco, J.J.; Joseph, T.; Clements, W. Immune function and the role of vaccination after splenic artery embolization for blunt splenic injury. *Injury* **2022**, *53*, 112–115. [CrossRef] [PubMed]
14. O'Rourke, C.; McKee, H.; Wijeyaratnam, D.O.; Bajwa, J.; Tremblay, L.; David, E. Retrospective Evaluation of Splenic Artery Embolization Outcomes in the Management of Blunt Splenic Trauma: A Single Centre Experience at a Large Level 1 Trauma Centre. *Can. Assoc. Radiol. J.* **2023**, *74*, 745–754. [CrossRef] [PubMed]
15. Yoo, R.; Evanson, D.; Gaziano, M.; Muller, A.; Martin, A.; Chauhan, N.; Butts, C.A.; Cortes, V.; Reilly, E.F.; Bamberger, P.K.; et al. Negative Splenic Angiography in Blunt Trauma: Does Embolization Affect Splenic Salvage? *Am. Surg.* **2023**, *89*, 3209–3211. [CrossRef] [PubMed]
16. Gasparetto, A.; Hunter, D.; Sapoval, M.; Sharma, S.; Golzarian, J. Splenic embolization in trauma: Results of a survey from an international cohort. *Emerg. Radiol.* **2021**, *28*, 955–963. [CrossRef] [PubMed]
17. Tidadini, F.; Martinet, E.; Quesada, J.-L.; Foote, A.; El Wafir, C.; Girard, E.; Arvieux, C.; SPLASH study group. Patient factors associated with embolization or splenectomy within 30 days of initiating surveillance for splenic trauma. *Emerg. Radiol.* **2024**, *31*, 823–833. [CrossRef] [PubMed]
18. Saba, G.B.; Rahal, R.; Bachir, R.; El Sayed, M. Factors associated with survival in adult trauma patients undergoing angiography with and without embolization across trauma centers in the United States. *Emerg. Radiol.* **2023**, *30*, 1–10. [CrossRef] [PubMed]
19. Nann, S.; Clark, M.; Kovoor, J.; Jog, S.; Aromataris, E. Prophylactic embolization vs observation for high-grade blunt trauma splenic injury: A systematic review with meta-analysis. *JBI Evid. Synth.* **2025**, *23*, 208–243. [CrossRef] [PubMed]
20. Arvieux, C.; Frandon, J.; Tidadini, F.; Monnin-Bares, V.; Foote, A.; Dubuisson, V.; Lermite, E.; David, J.-S.; Douane, F.; Tresallet, C.; et al. Effect of Prophylactic Embolization on Patients With Blunt Trauma at High Risk of Splenectomy: A Randomized Clinical Trial. *JAMA Surg.* **2020**, *155*, 1102–1111. [CrossRef] [PubMed] [PubMed Central]
21. Gill, K.; Aleman, S.; Fairchild, A.H.; Üstünsöz, B.; Laney, D.; Smith, A.A.; Ferral, H. Splenic artery embolization in the treatment of blunt splenic injury: Single level 1 trauma center experience. *Diagn. Interv. Radiol.* **2025**, *31*, 359–365. [CrossRef] [PubMed]
22. Lin, B.-C.; Wu, C.-H.; Wong, Y.-C.; Chen, H.-W.; Fu, C.-J.; Huang, C.-C.; Ku, Y.-K.; Chen, C.-C.; Sheng, T.-W.; Chang, C.-B. Comparison of outcomes of proximal versus distal and combined splenic artery embolization in the management of blunt splenic injury: A report of 202 cases from a single trauma center. *Surg. Endosc.* **2023**, *37*, 4689–4697. [CrossRef] [PubMed]
23. Stassen, N.A.; Bhullar, I.; Cheng, J.D.; Crandall, M.L.; Friese, R.S.; Guillamondegui, O.D.; Jawa, R.S.; Maung, A.A.; Rohs, T.J.; Sangosanya, A.; et al. Selective nonoperative management of blunt splenic injury: An Eastern Association for the Surgery of Trauma practice management guideline. *J. Trauma Acute Care Surg.* **2012**, *73* (Suppl. 4), S294–S300. [CrossRef] [PubMed]
24. American College of Surgeons Committee on Trauma. *Advanced Trauma Life Support (ATLS®) Student Course Manual*, 10th ed.; American College of Surgeons: Chicago, IL, USA, 2018.

Journal of
*Personalized Medicine*

MDPI

*Article*

# Efficacy and Safety of Personalized Percutaneous Single-Probe Cryoablation Using Liquid Nitrogen in the Treatment of Abdominal Wall Endometriosis

**Ghizlane Touimi Benjelloun [1,2,*], Malek Mokbli [1,2], Tarek Kammoun [1,2], Sinda Ghabri [1,2], Skander Sammoud [1,2], Wissem Nabi [1,2], Vincent Letouzey [3], Jean-Paul Beregi [1,2] and Julien Frandon [1,2]**

1 Department of Radiology and Medical Imaging, Nîmes University Hospital Center, University of Montpellier-Nîmes, 30900 Nîmes, France
2 Medical Imaging Group Nîmes (MIG Nîmes), 30900 Nîmes, France
3 Department of Gynecology and Obstetrics, Nîmes University Hospital Center, University of Montpellier-Nîmes, 30900 Nîmes, France
* Correspondence: ghizlane.touimibenjelloun@chu-nimes.fr

**Abstract: Background**: Abdominal wall endometriosis (AWE) is a rare but debilitating condition, often occurring in surgical scars after Caesarean sections. It is characterized by cyclic pain and a palpable mass, significantly impacting patients' quality of life. Traditional treatments, including hormonal therapy and surgery, have limitations, prompting interest in minimally invasive techniques such as cryoablation. This study evaluates the efficacy and safety of percutaneous image-guided single-probe cryoablation using liquid nitrogen for symptomatic AWE. **Purpose**: To evaluate the effectiveness and safety of percutaneous image-guided single-probe cryoablation using liquid nitrogen in treating symptomatic AWE lesions, with a primary objective to assess pain relief using the Visual Analog Scale (VAS). **Materials and Methods**: This retrospective, single-center study included 14 patients (23 lesions) treated with percutaneous cryoablation between September 2022 and April 2025. Clinical, imaging (MRI and ultrasound), and procedural data were analyzed. Pain scores (VAS scale) were assessed before treatment and at 3-month follow-up. Hydro- and/or carbo-dissection were used to protect adjacent structures. Response to treatment was evaluated with MRI and clinical follow-up. Statistical analysis was performed using median, range, and percentage calculations, with comparisons made using the Mann–Whitney test. **Results**: A total of 23 AWE lesions were treated in 14 patients (mean age: 39.6 years). The median lesion volume was 3546 mm$^3$, with a range from 331 mm$^3$ (8 × 4.6 × 9 mm) to 45,448 mm$^3$ (46 × 26 × 38 mm). Most of the lesions were located in the muscle (69.6%, $n$ = 16), while 17.4% ($n$ = 4) involved both muscle and subcutaneous tissue, and 13.0% ($n$ = 3) were purely subcutaneous. Among the 23 treated lesions, 8.7% ($n$ = 2) appeared as purely hemorrhagic, 13.0% ($n$ = 3) as fibrotic, and 78.3% ($n$ = 18) were classified as mixed, based on imaging characteristics. Procedures were performed under general anesthesia in 65% of cases and under sedation in 35%. Hydrodissection was used in 48% of lesions, carbo-dissection in 4%, and combined hydro–carbo dissection in 26%. A single 13G cryoprobe was used in 83% of cases, and a 10G probe in 17%. The median ablation time was 15 min (range: 6–28 min), and the median total procedure time was 93 min (range: 22–240 min). Pain scores significantly decreased from a median of 8/10 (range: 6–10) before treatment to 0/10 (range: 0–2) at follow-up ($p < 0.0001$). MRI follow-up confirmed complete coverage of the ablation zone and disappearance of hemorrhagic inclusions in all cases. Two patients (14%) required re-treatment, both with satisfactory outcomes. No peri- or post-procedural complications were observed, and no visible scars were noted. **Conclusions**: Percutaneous cryoablation using a single probe with liquid nitrogen is a safe and effective treatment for AWE, offering significant pain relief, minimal morbidity, and excellent cosmetic outcomes. It should be considered as part of multidisciplinary care. Further prospective studies with longer follow-up are warranted to confirm these findings.

**Keywords:** endometriosis; abdominal wall endometriosis; cryoablation; interventional radiology; single-probe; liquid nitrogen; pain

## 1. Introduction

Endometriosis is a chronic inflammatory condition that primarily affects young active women, particularly during their reproductive years, regardless of race or number of pregnancies. It is a leading cause of persistent pelvic pain, can significantly impact fertility, and adversely affects quality of life [1].

Abdominal wall endometriosis (AWE) is most commonly associated with surgical scars particularly following Caesarean sections. It is not always associated with deep pelvic endometriosis and often presents as an isolated condition. Patients typically experience cyclical symptom fluctuations, including pain and a palpable lump of the abdominal wall. Imaging techniques such as ultrasound and MRI are valuable tools for confirming the diagnosis [2–5].

Traditional treatment options for AWE to alleviate symptoms have been limited to hormonal therapies and extensive surgical interventions. However, recent studies have explored minimally invasive techniques to provide more localized symptom control. Cryoablation, in particular, has shown promise as a new treatment for AWE lesions, with favorable outcomes and low morbidity [6]. The visibility of ice formation on imaging allows for personalized treatment tailored to the size of the lesion and minimizes complications.

This single-center retrospective study aimed to assess the effectiveness and safety of percutaneous image-guided cryoablation with liquid nitrogen in treating symptomatic AWE. Our primary objective was to assess pain relief using VAS.

## 2. Materials and Methods

This observational, retrospective, monocentric non-interventional study was conducted between September 2022 and April 2025, involving 14 patients treated with single-probe percutaneous cryoablation using liquid nitrogen.

The study titled "Efficacy and Safety of Percutaneous Single Probe Cryoablation Using Liquid Nitrogen in the Treatment of Abdominal Wall Endometriosis" (ESCAWE) received a favorable opinion from the Institutional Review Board (Interface Recherche Bioéthique) of CHU Nîmes on 20 May 2025 (IRB Study Code: 25.05.01; Ref. No.: 35). The study is conducted in compliance with the General Data Protection Regulation (GDPR) and the French reference methodology MR004. All applicable ethical standards were adhered to, and an information and non-opposition note was provided in accordance with national regulations. Patients are free to refuse participation in the study after reviewing the information letter.

Patients are referred to us by their gynecologist or midwife. In some cases, the nodule is incidentally discovered on a pelvic MRI performed for the evaluation of pelvic pain. Our diagnostic radiology colleagues refer the patients to us, while also involving the hospital's gynecologists in the care pathway, and the choice to perform cryotherapy is made in a joint decision.

Patients were primarily selected for treatment due to pain, which was often described as severe. In rare cases, although the nodule was not painful, patients requested treatment either because they could feel a palpable mass or wished to discontinue hormonal therapy. For the purpose of this study, only patients treated for painful nodules were included.

Retrospectively, relevant demographic and clinical data were collected from medical records, prior consultations, procedural reports, and post-procedure follow-up at 3 months.

All patients underwent pelvic MRI using T2-weighted sequences, T1 gradient-echo multi-echo MR sequences (Dixon), diffusion-weighted sequences, and post-contrast T1-weighted sequences. The size, location (e.g., Caesarean scar, intramuscular, subcutaneous fat, peritoneal), and number of AWE target lesions were described. The lesion type (fibrotic, hemorrhagic, or mixed) was assessed based on MRI signal characteristics and post-contrast enhancement.

All patients were seen in consultation with an expert interventional radiologist, who evaluated pain using the VAS scale. Ultrasound was used to assess the accessibility of target lesions. Personalized treatment plans and potential complications were discussed during this consultation.

Written informed consent was obtained from all patients.

The approach to personalization primarily relied on procedural adaptation—including anesthesia choice, cryoprobe gauge, dissection techniques, and image guidance methods—based on lesion shape and size, location, patient anxiety, and imaging accessibility.

The novelty lies in the use of a single-probe cryoablation system. Indeed, this system enables us to go up to 4 cm iceball size, and we could relocate the cryoprobe to treat even bigger lesions.

Procedures were performed under general anesthesia or under sedation combined with local anesthesia. We are fortunate to collaborate daily with anesthesiologists in our operating room. Anesthesia protocols may vary between practitioners, and no standardized protocol is currently in place.

Before the treatment, the lesion was identified and measured under US guidance. Probe gauge (10G or 13G) was chosen depending on the lesion size and shape (two iceball shapes are available, round and elliptic). Hydro- and/or carbo-dissection were employed to protect the adjacent organs (digestive loops, bladder, nerves) and skin if they were at risk, using Chiba needles, placed under US or CT guidance.

We then performed freeze/passive thaw/freeze/active heat cycles, with equal duration of freeze and passive thaw cycles, depending on the size of the lesions and following the manufacturer's charts. The iceball was monitored all along the procedure under imaging guidance, and margins were assessed at the final control. Sometimes, probe relocation was needed if the nodule was too big.

Postoperatively, all patients were discharged the same day from the day hospital with well-controlled pain. A sick leave of 3 to 5 days was prescribed, along with nonsteroidal anti-inflammatory drugs (NSAIDs), level 1 analgesics, antiemetics, oral hydration, and laxatives if needed for constipation. Opioids were not required postoperatively for pain management.

Four to six weeks post-procedure, all patients underwent an MRI scan to evaluate for residual AWE lesions and potential complications. Pain and patient satisfaction were assessed during follow-up consultations at 3 months using the VAS scale and the aesthetic outcome.

Statistical analysis was performed using median, range, and percentage calculations, with comparisons made using the Mann–Whitney test. It was conducted with Microsoft Excel (Microsoft Corporation, Version 16.97.2).

This study was conducted for academic, non-profit purposes.

## 3. Results

The final sample consisted of 14 patients, with a mean age of 39.6 years, and a total of 23 ablated lesions. The median lesion volume was 3546 $mm^3$, with a range from 331 $mm^3$ (8 × 4.6 × 9 mm) to 45,448 $mm^3$ (46 × 26 × 38 mm). Of the lesions, 69.6% ($n$ = 16) were located in the muscle, 17.4% ($n$ = 4) involved both muscle and subcutaneous tissue, and 13.0% ($n$ = 3) were purely subcutaneous. Among the 23 treated lesions, 8.7% ($n$ = 2) were purely hemorrhagic, 13.0% ($n$ = 3) were fibrotic, and 78.3% ($n$ = 18) were classified as mixed, based on imaging characteristics. The hemorrhagic and mixed lesions displayed "powder burn" characteristics, appearing bright on T1 fat-saturated sequences (Figure 1).

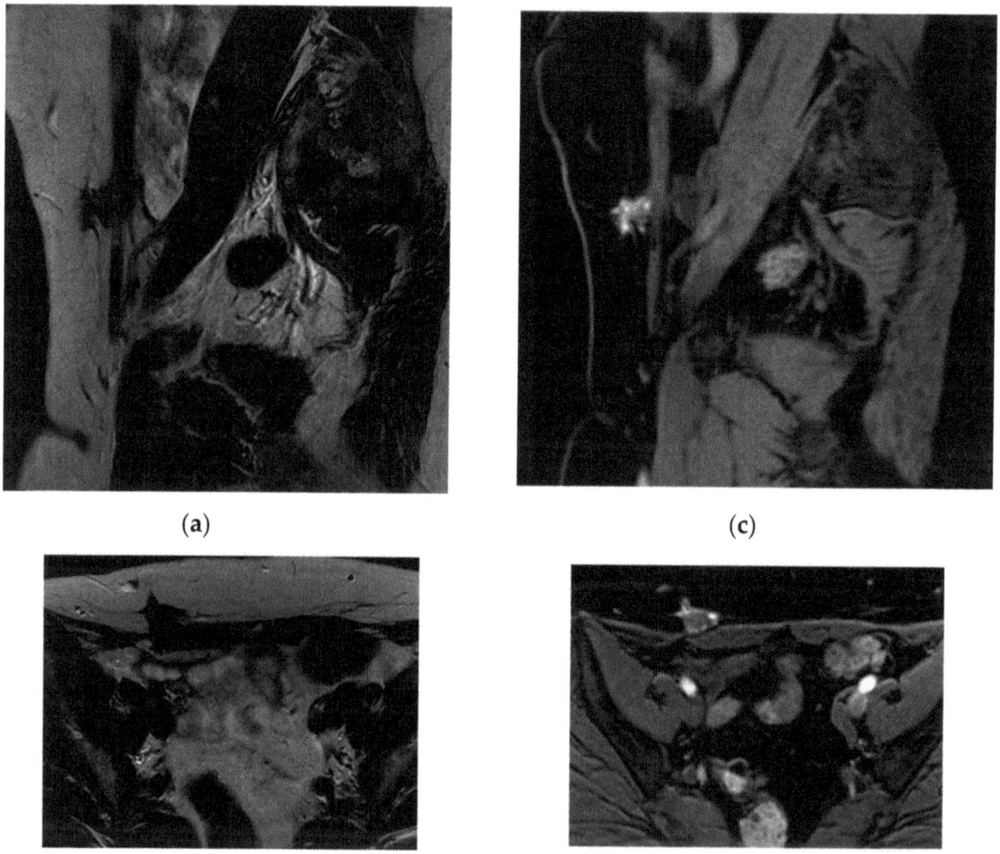

(a) (c)

(b) (d)

**Figure 1.** AWE on Caesarian section scar, developed in the subcutaneous fat without skin involvement, invading the underlying muscle, note the fibrous hyposignal on T2 WI (**a**,**b**) and hemorrhagic spots on T1 Water DIXON sequence (**c**,**d**).

Patient characteristics and lesion details are summarized in Table 1.

**Table 1.** Patient characteristics and lesion details.

| Number of Patients | 14 |
|---|---|
| Total Number of Lesions | 23 |
| Median Age | 39 years |
| Median Lesion Volume and Range | 3546 mm$^3$, with a range from 331 mm$^3$ (8 × 4.6 × 9 mm) to 45,448 mm$^3$ (46 × 26 × 38 mm). |
| Imaging Characteristics | - Mixed ($n$ = 18)<br>- Hemorrhagic ($n$ = 2)<br>- Fibrotic ($n$ = 3) |
| Lesion Locations | - Rectus abdominis muscle ($n$ = 16)<br>- Subcutaneous fat ($n$ = 3)<br>- Combined rectus abdominis + subcutaneous fat ($n$ = 4) |

The diagnosis of AWE was made based on clinical and imaging findings alone (US and MRI), which are both considered highly suggestive according to our experience and the literature. Therefore, no preoperative biopsy was performed for histological confirmation.

All patients were treated on an outpatient basis and were discharged the same day.

The treatment was performed under general anesthesia in 65% of cases ($n$ = 15) and under sedation in 35% ($n$ = 8). Hydrodissection was used in 48% of lesions ($n$ = 11), carbo-dissection in 4% ($n$ = 1), and hydro–carbo-dissection in 26% ($n$ = 6) to protect the digestive loops adjacent to the abdominal wall. Additionally, hydrodissection was used in 61% of cases ($n$ = 14) to protect the skin in superficial endometriotic lesions (Figure 2).

A single 13G cryoprobe was used in 83% of cases ($n$ = 19), and a 10G cryoprobe was used in 17% ($n$ = 4). The procedure was guided by ultrasound alone in 13% of cases ($n$ = 3), and by both CT and ultrasound in the remaining 87% ($n$= 20) to ensure accurate needle placement and iceball monitoring (Figure 3). Freeze–thaw–freeze cycles with active heating were applied, with a median ablation time of 15 min (range: 6–28 min), and a median total procedure time of 93 min (range: 22–240 min)

Two patients (14%) required re-treatment using the same modality. One was treated for persistent pain and a residual lesion on MRI, and the other for a new symptomatic AWE lesion occurring 13 months after the initial treatment. Both experienced satisfactory outcomes following re-treatment.

Pain significantly decreased from a median of 8/10 (range: 6–10) pre-procedure to 0/10 (range: 0–2) at last follow-up. A Mann–Whitney U test comparing VAS scores before and after cryoablation ($n$ = 19) showed a statistically significant reduction in pain, with a $p < 0.0001$. The MRI follow-up showed accurate targeting of the ablation zone, with complete coverage of the endometriotic nodule and disappearance of the hemorrhagic inclusions (Figure 4).

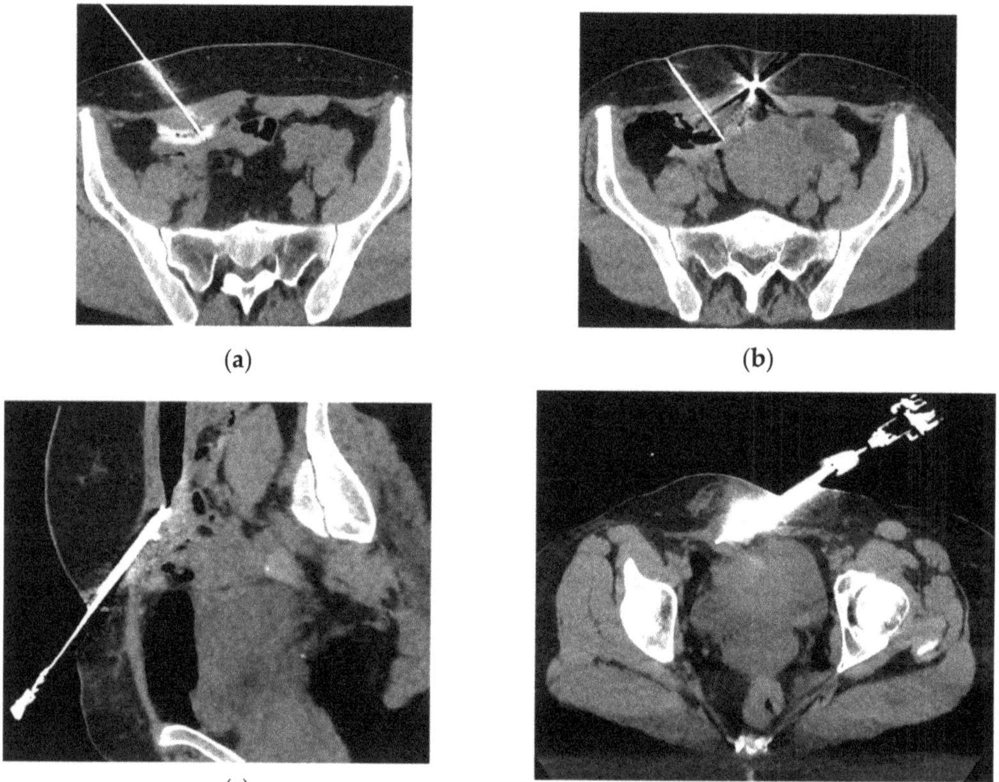

(a) (b) (c) (d)

**Figure 2.** Examples of protection techniques used to prevent damaging adjacent structures (skin and bowel): hydrodissection (**a**) or carbo-dissection (**b**,**c**) are performed after Chiba needle placement between the iceball and the sensitive organs to protect the bowel, and hydrodissection of the subcutaneous fat (**d**) to protect the skin.

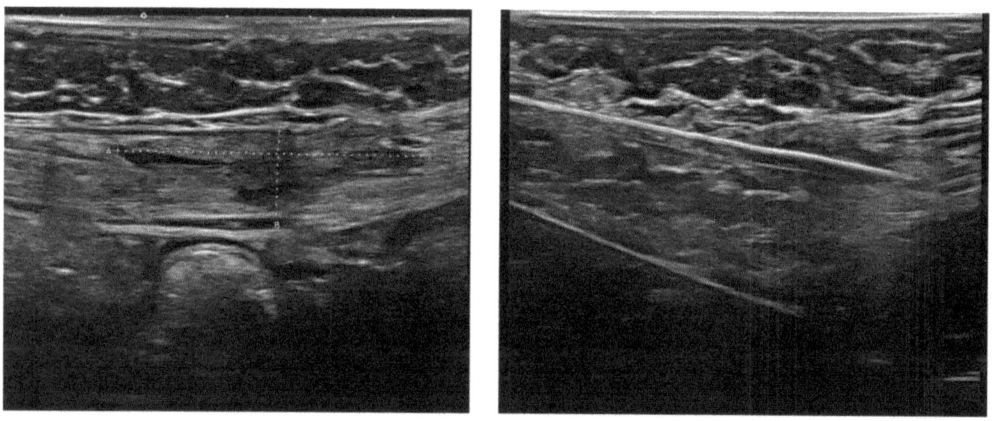

(a) (b)

**Figure 3.** *Cont.*

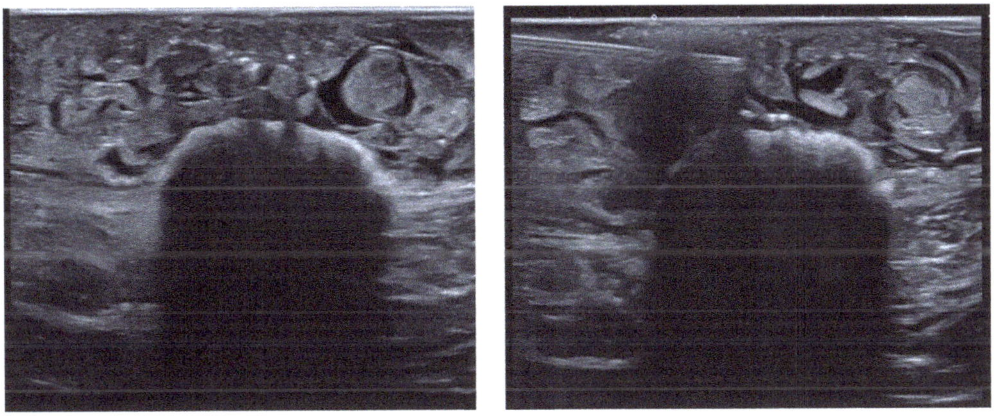

(c) (d)

**Figure 3.** Hypoechoic nodule of the rectus abdominis muscle (**a**) corresponding to AWE lesion. Cryoablation single-probe placement (**b**) and iceball monitoring under US guidance (**c**). Chiba Needle insertion under US guidance and Hydrodissection of the skin (**d**).

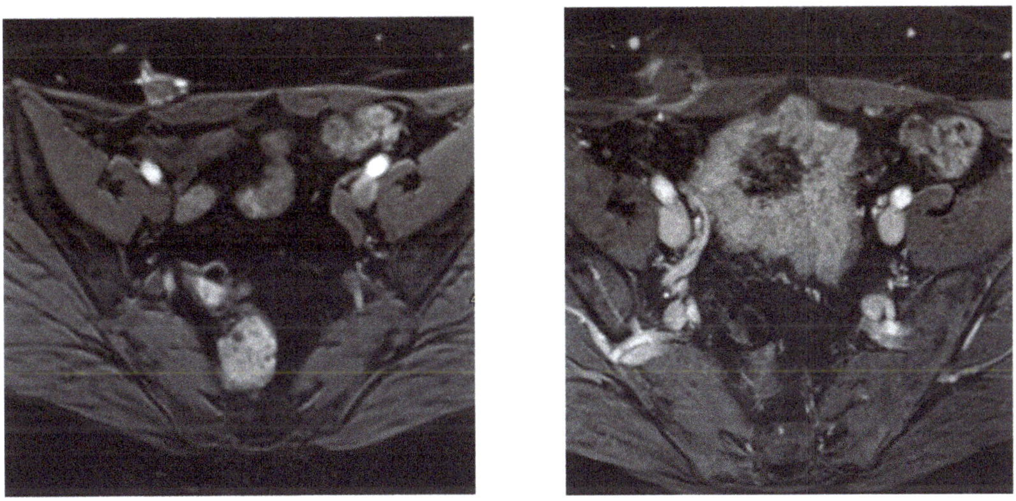

(a) (b)

**Figure 4.** Pre- (**a**) and post-cryoablation (**b**) MRI, contrast-enhanced T1 FS WI. On post-treatment MRI, we can notice the full coverage of the AWE lesion and an inflammatory rim enhancement, corresponding to a good imaging and clinical outcome.

## 4. Discussion

Abdominal wall endometriosis (AWE) is a rare manifestation of endometriosis, characterized by the presence of endometrial tissue within the abdominal wall, often at sites of previous surgical intervention. The incidence of AWE varies, with reports ranging from 0.03% to 3.5% among women undergoing abdominal surgeries, particularly cesarean sections [7].

Clinically, AWE typically presents as a palpable mass at or near surgical scars, accompanied by cyclic pain that correlates with the menstrual cycle. Patients often report localized discomfort or swelling in the affected area, which intensifies during menstruation. This pattern is considered pathognomonic for AWE [8].

The pathogenesis of AWE is believed to involve the direct implantation of endometrial cells into the abdominal wall during surgical procedures. These cells can proliferate and establish ectopic endometrial tissue, leading to the formation of endometriomas [7].

Given its rarity, AWE is frequently misdiagnosed, leading to significant diagnostic delays that can profoundly affect patients' psychological well-being. On average, individuals with endometriosis experience a diagnostic delay of approximately 8.6 years, which may lead to significant psychological distress, including anxiety and depression, as patients struggle with chronic pain and the lack of a definitive diagnosis [1].

In our cohort, one patient suffered from a diagnostic delay of 3 years since the onset of symptoms.

Abdominal wall endometriosis (AWE) presents with distinct imaging characteristics across various modalities, aiding in accurate diagnosis.

Ultrasound is often the first-line imaging modality for evaluating AWE. Lesions typically appear as solid, hypoechoic masses near surgical scars, such as those from cesarean sections. These masses may exhibit irregular or spiculated margins and can show vascularity on Doppler imaging. Occasionally, cystic changes are observed within the lesions [2].

CT imaging may reveal soft-tissue masses within the abdominal wall, often located near surgical scars. These masses can have irregular borders and may infiltrate adjacent tissues. However, CT is less specific than US and MRI for characterizing soft-tissue lesions like endometriosis [9].

MRI provides superior soft-tissue contrast, facilitating detailed assessment of AWE. Typically, on T1WI, lesions often exhibit hyperintense signals due to hemorrhagic content. On T2WI, lesions may show hypointense or heterogeneous signals, reflecting varying stages of hemorrhage and fibrosis. On contrast-enhanced T1WI, AWE lesions often exhibit enhancement reflecting vascularized endometrial tissue. This enhancement is variable and may not distinctly differentiate AWE from other benign or malignant processes. On DWI, AWE lesions can show hyperintensity with corresponding hypointensity on ADC maps, indicating restricted diffusion. This restriction is attributed to the dense cellularity and fibrotic components of the lesions. The mean ADC value of AWE has been reported as $0.93 \times 10^{-3}$ $mm^2/s$. These MRI characteristics are instrumental in differentiating AWE from other soft-tissue masses [3–5].

In our cohort, the imaging findings (US and MRI) matched the semiological features described in the literature.

In summary, integrating clinical history with imaging findings—such as hypoechoic masses on US and hyperintense signals on T1WI MRI—enhances the diagnostic accuracy for AWE. Thus, no pre-procedural biopsy was needed to confirm the diagnosis of AWE lesions in our patient cohort.

Cryoablation offers notable advantages over other ablative techniques in treating soft-tissue masses, including abdominal wall endometriosis (AWE), particularly concerning pain mitigation and aesthetic outcomes.

Indeed, cryoablation allows for precise visualization of the ablation zone. The ice-ball formed during the procedure is clearly delineated on imaging modalities such as ultrasound, CT, and MRI. This real-time monitoring facilitates accurate targeting and preservation of surrounding healthy tissues [10].

Furthermore, the cooling effect of cryoablation exerts an anesthetic property, leading to less procedural pain compared to heat-based methods like radiofrequency ablation (RFA) or microwave ablation (MWA). This often enables the use of local anesthesia and moderate sedation instead of general anesthesia [11]. In our cohort, both general anesthesia and sedation were used. The choice is adapted to each situation and depends on the evaluation of the radiologist, considering multiple parameters as the number and size of the lesions, the anxiety of the patient, and the complexity of the procedure.

Furthermore, Cornelis et al. reported that cryoablation led to substantial pain reduction and tumor size decrease in soft-tissue tumors, with a low incidence of severe adverse events [12]. In our study, pain decreased significantly from a median of 8/10 (range: 6–10) pre-procedure to 0/10 (range: 0–2) at last follow-up with $p < 0.0001$, and no peri- or post-operative adverse events were observed. These data confirm the efficacy and the safety of this technique.

Enhanced aesthetic outcomes are another advantage of percutaneous cryoablation. By minimizing damage to adjacent tissues and reducing inflammatory responses, cryoablation is associated with superior cosmetic results. This is particularly beneficial in treating superficial lesions where aesthetic considerations are paramount in a young female population [12,13]. In our patient cohort, no visible scar was observed.

One disadvantage of cryoablation is its longer procedural duration compared to microwave ablation (MWA) and radiofrequency ablation (RFA), as it requires at least two freeze cycles and one thaw cycle to achieve effective tissue destruction. This prolonged treatment time may be a consideration in clinical decision-making, particularly for larger lesions [14]. However, the small size of AWE lesions and the use of a single-probe technique minimize the impact of this longer treatment time. The median total procedure time in our cohort was 93 min, including patient setup and anesthesia time, which seems to be a reasonable duration.

Considering the cost-effectiveness of cryoablation as an alternative to surgical excision for treating AWE, although the initial expense of cryoprobes is relatively high, the overall cost of cryoablation can be lower than that of conventional surgery, depending on the country and the structure. A study comparing percutaneous cryoablation to surgery for extra-abdominal desmoid tumors—a condition with similarities to AWE—found that cryoablation resulted in cost savings, primarily due to reduced hospital stays and lower complication rates [15].

Single-probe cryoablation using liquid nitrogen adds another advantage to the technique compared to other cryoablation devices, as it is more cost-effective than those using Argon or Helium gas due to the large expense associated with their purchase and storage [14,16].

In the context of AWE, cryoablation has demonstrated similar effectiveness to surgery, with additional benefits such as shorter hospitalization and fewer complications. A study reported that patients undergoing cryoablation had a median hospital stay of 0.8 days compared to 2.8 days for those who underwent surgery. Additionally, 23.1% of surgical patients (3 out of 13 patients) experienced severe complications, whereas no severe complications were observed in the cryoablation group [12]. However, larger surgical studies report lower complication rates [17]. In our study, all patients were treated on an outpatient basis.

These factors contribute to the cost-effectiveness of cryoablation, offsetting the higher initial cost of cryoprobes and making it a financially viable option for AWE treatment.

In summary, cryotherapy treatment of parietal endometriosis lesions is planned in a personalized manner for each patient preoperatively, based on imaging characteristics (number, size, location, adjacent structures at risk) and the patient's profile. The final outcome is scar-free with significant clinical improvement, particularly regarding painful symptoms. These results confirm what has been reported in the literature about interventional radiology treatment of parietal endometriosis and reinforce the idea of moving toward less invasive, more precise medicine tailored to each situation.

Table 2 summarizes the findings of our study and the results of other published studies on cryoablation and/or surgery for AWE.

**Table 2.** Comparison between our study findings and other published studies on cryoablation or surgery for AWE.

| Study | Treatment Modality | Patients (n) | Median Follow-Up | Symptom-Free Rate at FU | Pain Reduction (VAS) | Aesthetic Outcome | Complications | Hospital Stay | Recurrence Rate |
|---|---|---|---|---|---|---|---|---|---|
| Touimi Benjelloun et al., 2025 | Cryoablation (single probe, liquid N2) | 14 (23 lesions) | 3 months | 86% (12/14) | 8→0 | No visible scar | None | Outpatient | 14% (2/14) |
| Maillot et al., 2017 [12] | Cryoablation vs. Surgery | 7 cryoablation/13 surgery | 22.5 months for cryoablation/ 54 months for surgery | 66.7% cryoablation/ 92% surgery | NR | No visible scan: cryoablation/69% aesthetic sequels: surgery | 0% cryoablation/ 23% surgery (severe complications) | 0.8 d cryoablation/2.8 d (surgery) | 14% cryoablation/7.7% surgery |
| Dibble et al., 2017 [11] | Cryoablation | 3 | 2.5 months | 2/3 patients | 8→0 | NR | None | Outpatient | NR |
| Najdawi et al., 2023 [18] | Cryoablation | 42 | 13.5 months | 82.72% | 8→0 | NR | 9.5% mild adverse events (skin burn); 2% severe adverse event (skin burn and small bowel injury) | Outpatient | 9.5% |
| Hasan et al., 2021 [19] | Surgical excision | 30 | 38 months (mean) | 100% (no recurrence) | VAS NR | NR | 33% (1 hernia, 5 wound infections, 4 bleedings) | Not reported | 0% |
| Horton et al., 2008 [20] | Surgical excision | 445 (445 lesions) | NR | 95% (symptom relief) | VAS NR | NR | NR | Not reported | 4.3% (Range 0% to 29%) |
| Benedetto et al., 2022 [17] | Surgical excision | 83 | US 6 mo after surgery + annual US | NR | Pre-op: 85% VAS $\leq$ 6, 15% $\geq$ 7; post-op: NR | NR | Hematoma/seroma 10.8%; Incisional Hernia 2.4%; (mostly > 30 mm lesions); no major events | 3 to 36 h (mean 16 h) | 0% |

This study, however, has several limitations that must be acknowledged. First, it is a retrospective, single-center study with a small sample size (14 patients, 23 lesions), which limits the statistical power and generalizability of the findings. The absence of a control group (e.g., surgical or medical management) prevents any direct comparison of cryoablation with standard treatment options.

Second, the follow-up period was limited to 3 months, which is insufficient to assess the long-term efficacy of cryoablation, recurrence rates, or durability of pain relief in a chronic and often recurrent condition such as endometriosis. This is an additional limitation of the retrospective study. In practice, patients return to their gynecologist for follow-up. In the event of symptom recurrence, they either contact us directly or are referred back by their gynecologist. A longer-term follow-up organized within interventional radiology is necessary to determine sustained outcomes and potential delayed complications.

Third, pain assessment relied exclusively on the VAS scale, which, while practical, remains subjective and susceptible to patient interpretation and reporting variability. No standardized quality-of-life questionnaires or functional outcomes were included.

These limitations highlight the need for prospective, multicenter studies with larger cohorts, standardized protocols, and longer follow-up to confirm the safety and effectiveness of cryoablation in the management of AWE.

## 5. Conclusions

In conclusion, percutaneous single-probe cryoablation using liquid nitrogen is an effective and safe treatment for AWE, particularly for younger patients, offering low post-operative morbidity and minimal adverse events. It is a viable alternative to traditional surgery, which typically involves general anesthesia, large surgical excisions, and considerable aesthetic damage.

Treatment decisions should be discussed in a multidisciplinary setting involving radiologists, interventional radiologists, and gynecologists. Future work should aim to define a more robust framework for personalized treatment of AWE, including clinical profiles, imaging features, and potentially biomarkers.

A 3-month follow-up is clearly insufficient to determine sustained outcomes in a chronic and recurrent condition such as endometriosis. Further cross-sectional studies and long-term follow-up organized within interventional radiology are necessary to fully assess the long-term results of this modality.

**Author Contributions:** Conceptualization, G.T.B. and J.F.; methodology, G.T.B. and T.K.; validation, G.T.B., J.F., J.-P.B. and V.L.; investigation, G.T.B., M.M. and S.G.; data curation, M.M. and S.S.; writing—original draft, G.T.B. and M.M.; writing—review and editing, G.T.B. and J.F.; visualization, G.T.B., M.M. and W.N. All authors have read and agreed to the published version of the manuscript.

**Funding:** This research received no external funding.

**Institutional Review Board Statement:** The study was reviewed and received favorable approval from the "Interface Recherche Bioéthique" Institutional Review Board (IRB) of CHU Nîmes on 20 May 2025 (Study Code: 25.05.01).

**Informed Consent Statement:** Informed consent was obtained from all subjects involved in the study.

**Data Availability Statement:** Dataset available on request from the authors.

**Conflicts of Interest:** The authors declare no conflicts of interest.

## References

1. Márki, G.; Vásárhelyi, D.; Rigó, A.; Kaló, Z.; Ács, N.; Bokor, A. Challenges of and possible solutions for living with endometriosis: A qualitative study. *BMC Womens Health* **2022**, 22, 20. [CrossRef] [PubMed]
2. Hensen, J.-H.J.; Van Breda Vriesman, A.C.; Puylaert, J.B.C.M. Abdominal Wall Endometriosis: Clinical Presentation and Imaging Features with Emphasis on Sonography. *Am. J. Roentgenol.* **2006**, 186, 616–620. [CrossRef] [PubMed]
3. Radzynski, L.; Boyer, L.; Kossai, M.; Mouraire, A.; Montoriol, P.-F. Pictorial essay: MRI evaluation of endometriosis-associated neoplasms. *Insights Imaging* **2023**, 14, 144. [CrossRef] [PubMed]
4. Hu, S.; Liu, Y.; Chen, R.; Xiao, Z. Exploring the Diagnostic Performance of Magnetic Resonance Imaging in Ultrasound-Guided High-Intensity Focused Ultrasound Ablation for Abdominal Wall Endometriosis. *Front. Physiol.* **2022**, 13, 819259. Available online: https://www.frontiersin.org/journals/physiology/articles/10.3389/fphys.2022.819259/full (accessed on 17 March 2025). [CrossRef] [PubMed]
5. Busard, M.P.H.; Mijatovic, V.; van Kuijk, C.; Hompes, P.G.A.; van Waesberghe, J.H.T.M. Appearance of abdominal wall endometriosis on MR imaging. *Eur. Radiol.* **2010**, 20, 1267–1276. [CrossRef] [PubMed]
6. Welch, B.T.; Ehman, E.C.; VanBuren, W.M.; Cope, A.G.; Welch, T.L.; Woodrum, D.A.; Kurup, A.N.; Burnett, T.L. Percutaneous cryoablation of abdominal wall endometriosis: The Mayo Clinic approach. *Abdom. Radiol.* **2020**, 45, 1813–1817. [CrossRef] [PubMed]
7. Encalada-Soto, D.; Zaucha, D.; Mikhail, E. Abdominal wall endometriosis: Pathogenesis, diagnosis, and update on minimally invasive treatment options: A narrative review. *Ann. Laparosc. Endosc. Surg.* **2023**, 10, 13. [CrossRef]
8. Foley, C.E.; Ayers, P.G.; Lee, T.T. Abdominal Wall Endometriosis. *Obstet. Gynecol. Clin.* **2022**, 49, 369–380. [CrossRef] [PubMed]
9. Stein, L.; Elsayes, K.M.; Wagner-Bartak, N. Subcutaneous Abdominal Wall Masses: Radiological Reasoning. *Am. J. Roentgenol.* **2012**, 198, W146–W151. [CrossRef] [PubMed]
10. Erinjeri, J.P. Overview of Thermal Ablation Devices: Cryoablation. In *Interventional Radiology Techniques in Ablation*; Clark, T., Sabharwal, T., Eds.; Springer: London, UK, 2013; pp. 13–19. [CrossRef]

11. Dibble, E.H.; D'Amico, K.C.; Bandera, C.A.; Littrup, P.J. Cryoablation of Abdominal Wall Endometriosis: A Minimally Invasive Treatment. *Am. J. Roentgenol.* **2017**, *209*, 690–696. [CrossRef] [PubMed]
12. Maillot, J.; Brun, J.L.; Dubuisson, V.; Bazot, M.; Grenier, N.; Cornelis, F.H. Mid-term outcomes after percutaneous cryoablation of symptomatic abdominal wall endometriosis: Comparison with surgery alone in a single institution. *Eur. Radiol.* **2017**, *27*, 4298–4306. [CrossRef] [PubMed]
13. Habrawi, Z.; Melkus, M.W.; Khan, S.; Henderson, J.; Brandi, L.; Chu, V.; Rahman, R.L. Cryoablation: A promising non-operative therapy for low-risk breast cancer. *Am. J. Surg.* **2021**, *221*, 127–133. [CrossRef] [PubMed]
14. Erinjeri, J.P.; Clark, T.W. Cryoablation: Mechanism of Action and Devices. *J. Vasc. Interv. Radiol.* **2010**, *21*, S187–S191. [CrossRef] [PubMed]
15. Narvaez, J.A.; Bernabeu, D.; Muntaner, L.; Gomez, F.; Martel, J.; Castellano, M.d.M.; García-Marcos, R.; Britel, R.; Oyagüez, I.; Tejado, N.; et al. Economic evaluation of percutaneous cryoablation vs conventional surgery in extra-abdominal desmoid tumours in the Spanish healthcare system. *Insights Imaging* **2024**, *15*, 1. [CrossRef] [PubMed]
16. Orsi, F.; Hamiddin, A.S.; Sattin, C.; Pizzi, C.; Varano, G.M.; Della Vigna, P.; Mauri, G.; Maiettini, D.; Bonomo, G. Liquid nitrogen-based cryoablation: Complication rates for lung, bone, and soft tissue tumors cryoablation. *Br. J. Radiol.* **2024**, *97*, 1863–1869. [CrossRef] [PubMed]
17. Benedetto, C.; Cacozza, D.; de Sousa Costa, D.; Coloma Cruz, A.; Tessmann Zomer, M.; Cosma, S.; Trippia, C.H.; Santos Cavalcanti, T.C.; Alves Castro, G.R.; Kondo, W. Abdominal wall endometriosis: Report of 83 cases. *Int. J. Gynecol. Obstet.* **2022**, *159*, 530–536. [CrossRef] [PubMed]
18. Najdawi, M.; Razakamanantsoa, L.; Mousseaux, C.; Bendifallah, S.; Touboul, C.; Thomassin-Naggara, I.; Bazot, M.; Barral, M.; Cornelis, F.H. Resolution of Pain after Percutaneous Image-Guided Cryoablation of Extraperitoneal Endometriosis. *J. Vasc. Interv. Radiol.* **2023**, *34*, 1192–1198. [CrossRef] [PubMed]
19. Hasan, A.; Deyab, A.; Monazea, K.; Salem, A.; Futooh, Z.; Mostafa, M.A.; Youssef, A.; Nasr, M.; Omar, N.; Rabaan, A.A.; et al. Clinico-pathological assessment of surgically removed abdominal wall endometriomas following cesarean section. *Ann. Med. Surg.* **2021**, *62*, 219–224. [CrossRef] [PubMed]
20. Horton, J.D.; DeZee, K.J.; Ahnfeldt, E.P.; Wagner, M. Abdominal wall endometriosis: A surgeon's perspective and review of 445 cases. *Am. J. Surg.* **2008**, *196*, 207–212. [CrossRef] [PubMed]

Journal of *Personalized Medicine*

MDPI

*Article*

# Prostate Artery Embolization (PAE) with Small Beads for the Treatment of Benign Prostatic Hyperplasia (BPH)

**Genti Xhepa [1,2,*], Lucilla Violetta Sciacqua [3], Andrea Vanzulli [3,4], Andrea Enzo Cani [5], Velio Ascenti [3], Alexis Ricoeur [2], Andrea Antonio Ianniello [6], Agostino Inzerillo [7], Paolo Nicotera [8], Filippo Del Grande [1,9], Anna Maria Ierardi [10] and Gianpaolo Carrafiello [10]**

1 Istituto di Imaging della Svizzera Italiana (IIMSI), Ente Ospedaliero Cantonale (EOC), 6900 Lugano, Switzerland; filippo.delgrande@eoc.ch
2 Interventional Radiology Unit, University Hospital of Geneva (HUG), 1205 Geneva, Switzerland; alexis.ricoeur@hcuge.ch
3 Postgraduate School in Radiodiagnostics, University of Milan, 20122 Milan, Italy; lucilla.sciacqua@unimi.it (L.V.S.); andrea.vanzulli@unimi.it (A.V.); velio.ascenti@unimi.it (V.A.)
4 Department of Radiology, Fondazione IRCCS Istituto Nazionale dei Tumori di Milano, 20133 Milan, Italy
5 Department of Diagnostic and Interventional Radiology, Ospedale di Garbagnate Milanese "Guido Salvini", ASST Rhodense, 20024 Garbagnate Milanese, Italy; aecani@asst-rhodense.it
6 Department of Radiology, Luigi Sacco University Hospital, 20157 Milan, Italy; ianniello.andrea@asst-fbf-sacco.it
7 AOUP Paolo Giaccone, Biomedicine, Neuroscience and Advanced Diagnostic Department (BiND), University of Palermo, 90127 Palermo, Italy; inzerilloagostino@gmail.com
8 Radiology Unit, Ospedale di Circolo e Fondazione Macchi, University of Insubria, 21100 Varese, Italy; paolonicotera78@gmail.com
9 Facoltà di Scienze Biomediche, Campus Est, Università Della Svizzera Italiana (USI), 6900 Lugano, Switzerland
10 Department of Radiology, Foundation IRCCS Ca' Granda-Ospedale Maggiore Policlinico, University of Milan, 20122 Milan, Italy; anna.ierardi@unimi.it (A.M.I.); gianpaolo.carrafiello@unimi.it (G.C.)
* Correspondence: genti_xh@hotmail.com or genti.xhepa@eoc.ch; Tel.: +41-794748431

**Abstract:** Benign Prostatic Hyperplasia (BPH) is the most frequent cause of Lower Urinary Tract Symptoms (LUTSs) in elderly populations. Minimally invasive treatments of BPH are safe and effective and are gaining popularity among both professionals and patients. Prostate Artery Embolization (PAE) has proven to be effective in Trans-Urethral Resection of the Prostate (TURP) in terms of prostate volume reduction and LUTS relief. PAE entails the selective catheterization of the prostatic artery and later embolization of distal vessels with beads of various calibers. Universal consensus regarding the ideal particle size is yet to be defined. We retrospectively evaluated 24 consecutive patients (median age: 75 years; range: 59–86 years) treated with PAE at our institution from October 2015 to November 2022. Particles of different sizes were employed; 12 patients were treated with 40–120 μm particles, 5 with 100 μm, 5 with 100–300 μm and 2 with 250 μm. Technical success, defined as selective prostate artery catheterization and controlled release of embolizing beads, was achieved in all patients. Removal vs. retention of the urinary catheter at the first post-procedural urological visit was the main clinical objective. No major peri-procedural complications were recorded, with 56% of patients successfully removing the urinary catheter.

**Keywords:** Benign Prostatic Hyperplasia; Lower Urinary Tract Symptoms; Prostate Artery Embolization; urinary catheter; interventional radiology

## 1. Introduction

Benign Prostatic Hyperplasia (BPH) represents a non-neoplastic condition characterized by aberrant cellular proliferation within the transitional zone (TZ) of the prostate gland. The escalating prevalence and incidence of BPH have been robustly associated with advancing age demographics [1]. Recent scholarly inquiries have delineated a panoply of modifiable risk factors intricately involved in the genesis of early-stage BPH. These encompass serum dihydrotestosterone (DHT) concentrations, adiposity indices, glucose homeostasis perturbations, dietary constituents, physical activity regimens, and inflammatory mediators [1–4].

Autopsy-derived epidemiological data delineate a progressive increase in the prevalence of BPH with advancing age, standing at 8% in the fourth decade, escalating to 50% in the sixth decade, and peaking at 80% in the ninth decade [1]. This condition presents formidable clinical challenges, particularly as it predominantly afflicts elderly individuals burdened with a plethora of coexisting medical conditions [1]. BPH emerges as the principal instigator of Lower Urinary Tract Symptoms (LUTSs), afflicting an estimated 70% of males beyond the age of 80 [5]. LUTS, characterized by their incapacitating nature, exert a significant toll on the quality of life for those affected. The assessment of LUTS impact commonly relies on the International Prostate Symptom Score (IPSS), a validated tool employed to discern the extent of symptomatology's intrusion into daily activities [6].

Acute Urinary Retention (AUR) stands out as the most critical complication associated with BPH, constituting a life-threatening event that ensues in up to 10% of men aged 70–79 diagnosed with BPH [7,8].

AUR mandates immediate intervention to alleviate obstruction, typically through catheterization, as its unmitigated progression poses a significant risk of precipitating acute renal injury [9,10]. Symptomatic BPH engenders a diverse array of therapeutic strategies for effective management.

In accordance with the guidelines set forth by the European Association of Urology (EAU), initial interventions for LUTS attributed to BPH predominantly center on medical interventions and lifestyle adjustments [11]. Implementation of straightforward behavioral modifications, such as restricting evening fluid intake, holds promise in attenuating the frequency of nocturia. Additionally, the avoidance of diuretic agents and incorporation of pelvic floor exercises present viable strategies for mitigating urinary frequency, a pivotal component of the IPSS [11].

The utilization of alpha 1-adrenoceptor antagonists ($\alpha$1-blockers), either as monotherapy or in conjunction with 5-alpha reductase inhibitors (5-ARIs), stands as a cornerstone in alleviating BPH-related symptoms [12]. However, in instances where primary interventions prove inadequate or elicit intolerable adverse effects, surgical intervention becomes imperative.

According to the latest guidelines, transurethral resection of the prostate (TURP) remains the gold standard surgical intervention for managing BPH [13–15]. TURP involves the meticulous insertion of a resectoscope through the penile urethra, targeting the central prostatic region responsible for symptomatic presentation. This procedure aims to effectuate rapid de-obstruction. Both bipolar (b-TURP) and monopolar (m-TURP) techniques are commonly employed and yield comparable outcomes in terms of symptom relief. However, b-TURP often demonstrates superior efficacy and is associated with lower complication rates, particularly in cases involving larger prostates [16,17].

Key complications reported with TURP encompass clot retention (2–5%), necessitating post-procedure blood transfusions (0.4–7.1%), urinary tract infections (1.7–8.2%), and less frequent occurrences of TUR syndrome (0–1.1%). TUR syndrome arises from the absorption of electrolyte-free irrigating fluid and represents a potentially serious complication of the procedure [18–21].

Notwithstanding the considerable success of TURP in managing BPH, the potential for complications or contraindications has instigated the exploration of innovative, minimally invasive therapeutic avenues.

The introduction of laser-based prostate enucleation techniques has emerged as a significant development, notably featuring holmium laser enucleation of the prostate (HoLEP) and thulium laser enucleation of the prostate (ThuLEP) as prominent modalities [18]. Comparative investigations between HoLEP and TURP have underscored several advantages associated with HoLEP, including abbreviated hospitalization durations, reduced periods of catheterization, and augmented hemostatic capabilities, thereby mitigating bleeding-related complications. However, HoLEP typically entails a lengthier operative duration, primarily attributable to the additional morcellation time necessitated [22–27].

Within the realm of Minimally Invasive Surgical Therapies (MISTs), Prostatic Urethral Lift (PUL) and Water Vapor Thermal Therapy (WVTT), also known as Rezum, have garnered attention as promising alternatives, exhibiting notable efficacy in ameliorating urinary symptoms among treated individuals [28,29]. The PUL technique involves the deployment of the UroLift Device, which releases small permanent implants to mechanically widen the prostatic urethra, thereby alleviating symptomatic obstruction [30]. Conversely, WVTT represents an outpatient procedure leveraging radiofrequency technology. Here, a transurethral device administers water steam to the prostate's transition zone, inducing coagulative necrosis within the treated area [31,32].

Innovative minimally invasive techniques have emerged as pivotal adjuncts in the therapeutic armamentarium for BPH, encompassing ablative methodologies such as Transurethral Needle Ablation (TUNA), Transurethral Microwave Ablation (TUMT), and partial cryoablation [33–38]. Following the insertion of specialized devices into the urethra, these techniques achieve coagulative necrosis of prostatic tissue, employing either radiofrequencies (as in TUNA) or microwaves (as in TUMT).

The absence of a universally superior minimally invasive modality underscores the complexity of BPH management [15,16,31]. Factors including prostate volume, risk of sexual dysfunction, surgical risk, and patient preferences collectively inform the selection of the most appropriate treatment modality for individual patients [16,18].

According to the Society of Interventional Radiology (SIR), Prostate Artery Embolization (PAE) represents a viable therapeutic avenue for addressing LUTS attributed to BPH, exhibiting comparable efficacy to surgical interventions [16,39–42]. The allure of PAE is further accentuated by its associated benefits, including reduced hospitalization durations, diminished transfusion risks, and a low incidence of sexual dysfunction [16,41,43].

Initially relegated to emergency scenarios such as hemorrhage, PAE has demonstrated remarkable efficacy in reducing prostate volume, albeit with delayed onset of action and fewer procedure-related risks compared to surgical interventions [44]. Presently, PAE emerges as an optimal strategy for patients unsuitable for surgery, those averse to surgical interventions, or individuals prioritizing the preservation of sexual function [16,40].

The primary risk associated with PAE pertains to non-target embolization, with unfavorable vascular anatomy serving as a principal contraindication to the procedure [43]. Selective catheterization of prostate arteries is facilitated through microcatheters or microguides, followed by occlusion employing various embolic agents. Spherical polyvinyl alcohol (PVA) particles of varying diameters, notably within the ranges of 100–300 µm, 250–400 µm, or 300–500 µm, constitute the predominant embolic agents employed [45–47]. The optimal bead caliber remains a subject of ongoing discourse [48,49].

In the study conducted by Bilhim et al., a meticulous examination of the embolic particle size's impact on the efficacy and safety profile of PAE was undertaken [49]. Their findings unveiled a nuanced interplay between particle size and clinical outcomes, delineating distinct advantages and limitations associated with different particle sizes.

Notably, larger embolic particles (>200 µm) exhibited superior clinical outcomes in subjective parameters such as the International Prostate Symptom Score (IPSS) and peak flow rate (Qmax) [49]. Conversely, smaller particles demonstrated enhanced efficacy in objective parameters, particularly in reducing Prostate-Specific Antigen (PSA) levels [49]. This dichotomy in efficacy can be attributed to the deeper penetration of smaller particles into the distal prostatic arteries, inducing a more extensive area of ischemia and subsequent prostate shrinkage.

However, this apparent advantage of smaller particles in reducing prostate volume was tempered by concerns regarding increased side effects reported in some early studies [47]. This phenomenon was hypothesized to result from the deeper penetrating nature of smaller particles, potentially predisposing them to enter anastomotic arterial vessels and lead to non-target embolization.

Nevertheless, Bilhim et al.'s investigation provided reassurance by demonstrating that there were no significant differences in adverse events following PAE with 100 μm or 200 μm PVA particles [49]. This observation suggests a potential equilibrium between therapeutic efficacy and safety across different particle sizes.

In our own study, we aimed to extend these findings by evaluating the response to PAE treatment utilizing particles of varying diameters in a cohort of patients affected by LUTSs attributable to BPH. Additionally, we sought to comprehensively analyze the occurrence of potential complications associated with different particle sizes.

Our assessment of treatment response was predicated on the retention or removal of the bladder catheter, serving as a clinically relevant indicator of treatment efficacy and patient comfort.

## 2. Materials and Methods

In our retrospective study, we analyzed a cohort consisting of 24 consecutive patients, with a median age of 75 years (range: 59–86 years), who underwent PAE utilizing beads of various sizes (ranging from 40 to 300 μm) at our medical institution between October 2015 and November 2022.

Before the initiation of treatment, the cohort exhibited an average prostate volume of 116.5 mL, with prostate volumes ranging from 26 mL in cases previously managed with TURP to a maximum of 309 mL. Notably, all patients had a dependency on indwelling urinary catheters due to antecedent episodes of AUR attributed to the presence of large central adenomas. Additionally, one patient presented with persistent hematuria.

Inclusion criteria for enrollment in this study were based on the absence of prostate cancer or other neoplastic pathologies, favorable anatomical suitability for PAE, and documented failure of initial-line therapeutic interventions, as delineated in Table 1.

**Table 1.** Inclusion and exclusion criteria for patients receiving PAE in our study.

| Exclusion Criteria | Inclusion Criteria |
|---|---|
| Prostate cancer | Favourable anatomy |
| Synchronous tumours | Failure of first-line therapy |
| Pseudoaneurysm | Presence of permanent catheter |
| Penile anastomosis | Contraindications to TURP |
| | Patients' choice |

Two patients subjected to PAE had previously undergone surgical intervention via TURP, but experienced a recurrence of AUR necessitating catheter repositioning. Intraoperative assessment of vascular anatomy feasibility was conducted via arteriography.

Exclusion criteria were applied to the following three patients: one presenting with synchronous bladder cancer, another necessitating coil deployment instead of beads to address a bleeding pseudoaneurysm, and a third case in which embolization was aborted due to the presence of a contraindication (penile anastomosis) detected during intraprocedural imaging. Additionally, two patients were excluded due to PAE procedures utilizing both small and large particles (one treated with 100–300 μm and 40–120 μm, and the other with 100 μm and 300–500 μm particles).

In all instances, super-selective catheterization of prostatic arteries was meticulously performed using microcatheters to minimize the risk of non-target embolization. The correct positioning of microcatheters was meticulously verified utilizing Cone Beam Computed Tomographic Angiography (CBCTA), as exemplified in Figure 1.

PAE was performed under local anesthesia using the unilateral approach in 8 patients or the bilateral femoral approach in 16 patients, using particles with different sizes in a range between 40 μm and 300 μm; 12 patients were treated with 40–120 μm particles, 5 patients with 100 μm, 5 patients with 100–300 μm and 2 patients with 250 μm.

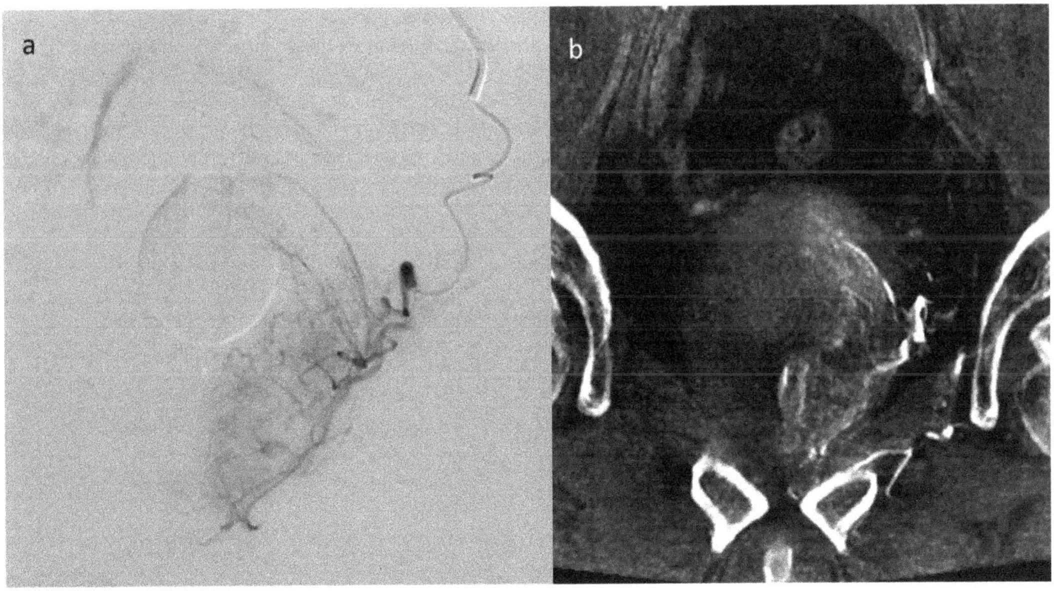


**Figure 1.** (**a**) Superselective Digital Subtraction Angiography (DSA) and (**b**) Cone Beam Computed Tomographic Angiography (CBCTA) of the left prostate artery.

## 3. Results

Technical success, defined as super-selective catheterization of the prostate artery and the controlled release of embolizing beads, was achieved in all patients. For the evaluation of complications, we considered the latest updated classification of adverse events (AEs) proposed by the Society of Interventional Radiology (SIR) [50,51]. Considering every scenario contemplated by the SIR, no major procedure-related complications were registered. Additionally, there were no cases of increased hospitalization.

The clinical evaluation was performed for only a few patients by using the IPSS questionnaire, as most of them were outpatients, followed outside the hospital. Therefore, we did not take the IPSS into consideration in the final evaluation of our work.

The primary clinical outcome measured was the removal of the urinary catheter at the first post-procedural follow-up.

At follow-up intervals of 6 months and 1 year, the outcomes related to urinary catheter use were assessed across all patients, irrespective of the particle size used in the procedure. Only one patient did not require catheter placement immediately after the procedure due to effective urination with no post-void residuals (PVRs). In contrast, 56% of patients were able to remove the catheter at their first post-procedural visit, even when presenting with minimal or non-pathological PVR. However, one patient required catheter repositioning one month after the procedure due to a relapse of AUR. Additionally, 20% of patients were unable to remove the catheter after PAE due to high PVR levels.

When analyzing outcomes based on the size of the embolizing particles, the following observations were made: among the twelve patients treated with the smallest particles (40–120 μm), one patient did not require bladder catheterization, nine patients removed the catheter at the first post-procedural visit, and one patient needed catheter repositioning one month after PAE due to recurrence of AUR.

Among the five patients treated with 100 μm particles, two were successful in removing the catheter, two required continued catheter use, and one patient needed a ureterocutaneostomy due to persistent hematuria, which was unrelated to the procedure.

Of the five patients treated with 100–300 μm particles, three were able to remove the catheter at the first post-procedural visit, while two needed to maintain catheter use.

Patients treated with 250 μm particles were all unsuccessful in removing the catheter following the procedure.

A comparative analysis of patient outcomes based on the size of embolizing particles used during PAE revealed significant differences in the success rates of catheter removal. In the group treated with smaller particles (40–120 μm and 100 μm), 70.6% of patients were able to successfully remove their catheter. Conversely, in the group treated with larger particles (100–300 μm and 250 μm), only 42.9% of patients achieved successful catheter removal. Furthermore, patients who were able to remove their catheters did not exhibit any PVR or pathological urinary residue.

Notably, all patients who successfully removed their catheters after the procedure did not experience any recurrence of AUR at the 1-year follow-up mark.

PAE results with different particle sizes are presented in Table 2.

**Table 2.** Results in terms of CV removal–retention and PVR of patients treated with PAE with beads stratified by size.

| Patient# | Particles Caliber | Access | Outcome | PVR |
|---|---|---|---|---|
| 1 | 40–120 | Bilat | No CV | No |
| 2 | 40–120 | R | Removal CV | No |
| 3 | 40–120 | Bilat | Removal CV | 130 mL |
| 4 | 40–120 | Bilat | Removal CV | Non-pathological |
| 5 | 40–120 | Bilat | Removal CV | Non-pathological |
| 6 | 40–120 | Bilat | Removal CV | No |
| 7 | 40–120 | Bilat | Removal CV | No |
| 8 | 40–120 | L | Removal CV | Non-pathological |
| 9 | 40–120 | Bilat | Removal CV | No |
| 10 | 40–120 | Bilat | Removal CV | No |
| 11 | 40–120 | Bilat | Repositioning after 1 month | Relapse of AUR |
| 12 | 40–120 | L | Removal CV | 102 mL |
| 13 | 100 | R | Removal CV | No |
| 14 | 100 | L | Removal CV | No |
| 15 | 100 | Bilat | Retention of CV | High |
| 16 | 100 | R | Retention of CV | High |
| 17 | 100 | L | Ureterocutaneostomy | Haematuria |
| 18 | 100–300 | Bilat | Removal CV | No |
| 19 | 100–300 | Bilat | Removal CV | No |
| 20 | 100–300 | Bilat | Removal CV | No |
| 21 | 100–300 | L | Retention of CV | High |
| 22 | 100–300 | Bilat | Retention of CV | High |
| 23 | 250 | Bilat | Retention of CV | High |
| 24 | 250 | Bilat | Retention of CV | Haematuria |

In assessing prostate size before and after treatment, data from 17 cases were analyzed to derive prostate volumes at either the 6-month or 1-year post-operative follow-up. Across the cohort, a consistent decrease in gland volume was observed, except for one patient treated with small particles (40–120 μm) who exhibited no change in prostate volume.

When examining the total number of patients treated with small particles (diameters 40–120 μm and 100 μm), an average reduction in prostate volume of 76% was noted. This reduction was comparable to the average reduction of 75.6% observed among patients undergoing PAE with larger particles (100–300 μm and 250 μm).

Despite the differences in patient group sizes and the lack of statistical significance, it is noteworthy that the average post-procedural reduction in prostate volume was similar between the two groups. This observation suggests a consistent efficacy of PAE across varying particle sizes, albeit with variations in individual patient responses.

## 4. Discussion

As global life expectancy continues its upward trajectory, the prevalence of LUTS attributed to BPH escalates, especially among men aged 60 and above. These symptoms, often severe and refractory to initial pharmacological interventions, present formidable clinical challenges. Despite optimized medical management, a significant subset of patients continues to experience persistent LUTS, necessitating more invasive interventions [1]. Transurethral resection of the prostate (TURP) remains the gold standard for such cases, yet it carries inherent risks, including intra- and post-procedural bleeding, infection, and the potential for TUR syndrome [15,18,21]. However, certain patients pose complexities due to the presence of multiple comorbidities or contraindications to surgery, prompting the exploration of alternative interventions that offer comparable efficacy to TURP but with reduced invasiveness.

The clinical dilemma is particularly acute when dealing with prostates exceeding 100 mL in volume, as the risks associated with TURP, such as heightened intraoperative and perioperative complications and extended recovery periods, become magnified [52]. In response to these challenges, modalities utilizing holmium (HoLEP) or thulium (ThuLEP) lasers have emerged as promising alternatives. These techniques have demonstrated substantial efficacy in reducing prostate volume while conferring several advantages over conventional TURP, including shorter hospital stays, improved hemostasis, and lower complication rates [22,23,27].

As such, there is a burgeoning interest within the medical community in exploring these less invasive approaches as viable strategies for managing BPH-related LUTS, particularly among patient populations with heightened surgical risks or preferences for minimally invasive interventions. This underscores the imperative for further research and clinical evaluation to ascertain the optimal treatment paradigm for this challenging patient cohort.

The PUL technique has emerged as a subject of considerable interest owing to its notable efficacy, particularly in addressing the intricate challenges presented by larger prostatic volumes. This innovative approach involves the strategic application of tension to the prostatic lobes, thereby inducing compression of the prostatic urethra [30,53].

It has been demonstrating that WVTT, also known as Rezum, is very effective in IPSS improvement and it has shown a significant decrease in the bladder outlet obstruction index (BOOI). Both young and elderly patients can benefit from this technique because of its short operative time [54]. Moreover, ongoing research endeavors underscore the burgeoning evidence supporting the efficacy of WVTT in ameliorating LUTS associated with prostates exceeding the volumetric threshold of 80 cm$^3$ [55].

Furthermore, laser-based modalities have demonstrated noteworthy efficacy in the management of larger prostatic volumes [56].

In stark contrast, ablative interventions such as TUNA and TUMT offer immediate reductions in prostatic volume. However, their efficacy tends to diminish when confronted with larger prostates [16,52].

Conversely, PAE has emerged as a compelling therapeutic avenue for the management of LUTS attributed to BPH. PAE not only yields outcomes akin to those achieved through TURP but also mitigates operative risks [39–42]. A salient advantage of PAE is its adaptability to prostates exceeding the volumetric threshold of 100 mL, with consistently favorable clinical outcomes [57].

The main controversy remains in the choice of embolizing particle size [48,49,58].

Some studies support that large particles are more effective in clinical improvement as assessed by IPSS, while smaller particles act more markedly on the reduction in objective parameters, such as PSA [49].

Regarding adverse events, Bilhim et al. demonstrated that there are no significant differences in adverse events after PAE with 100 μm or 200 μm PVA particles, while Wang et al. stated that there are no significant differences between the use of 50–100 μm particles or 100 μm PVA particles alone [49,58].

The central point of contention within the field of PAE revolves around the selection of embolizing particle size, a topic extensively scrutinized in the literature [48,49,58]. Various studies have contributed to this discourse, presenting divergent perspectives on the efficacy of different particle sizes in achieving clinical improvement and mitigating adverse events.

One line of inquiry suggests that larger embolizing particles may yield superior clinical outcomes, particularly evident in the amelioration of symptoms as assessed by the IPSS [49]. Conversely, smaller particles appear to exert a more pronounced effect on objective parameters such as PSA levels, thus highlighting potential nuances in the therapeutic mechanisms of different particle sizes [49].

The assessment of adverse events further complicates this matter, with studies yielding conflicting findings regarding the comparative safety profiles of different particle sizes. For instance, Bilhim et al. found no significant disparities in adverse event rates following PAE with either 100 µm or 200 µm polyvinyl alcohol (PVA) particles [49]. In contrast, Wang et al. reported similar outcomes between the use of 50–100 µm particles and 100 µm PVA particles alone [58]. These contrasting findings underscore the complexity of the relationship between particle size and procedural safety, necessitating further investigation to elucidate optimal strategies for minimizing adverse events during PAE.

Our study provides detailed insights into the outcomes of prostatic artery embolization (PAE), particularly concerning the influence of embolizing particle size. We achieved a high rate of technical success, with all patients undergoing super-selective catheterization of the prostate artery and controlled release of embolizing beads. This success was observed across all patients, regardless of the embolizing particle size used during the procedure. Furthermore, no major procedure-related complications according to the SIR Classification were noted in any of the patients, aligning with previous research indicating PAE as a safe and effective procedure for managing BPH [50,51].

In terms of clinical outcomes, our study revealed variations in catheter removal success rates following PAE. Among the patients treated with smaller particles (40–120 µm and 100 µm), a higher proportion successfully removed the catheter compared to those treated with larger particles (100–300 µm and 250 µm). Specifically, 70.6% of patients treated with smaller particles successfully removed their catheters, while only 42.9% of patients treated with larger particles achieved successful catheter removal. Notably, the success rates varied depending on the embolizing particle size used, suggesting a potential influence of particle size on clinical outcomes such as catheter removal success.

When comparing our findings to existing literature, we observed conflicting evidence regarding adverse event rates associated with different particle sizes in PAE. Bilhim et al. found no significant differences in adverse event rates between procedures utilizing 100 µm and 200 µm polyvinyl alcohol (PVA) particles [49], while Wang et al. reported similar outcomes between procedures utilizing 50–100 µm particles and those utilizing 100 µm PVA particles alone [58]. These discrepancies underscore the complexity of the relationship between particle size and procedural safety, highlighting the need for further investigation to elucidate optimal strategies for minimizing adverse events during PAE.

While our study sheds some light on the outcomes of PAE, there are several limitations that need to be acknowledged.

Firstly, the study's sample size was relatively small, potentially limiting the generalizability of the findings. Secondly, the retrospective design of the study introduces inherent biases and limitations associated with retrospective data collection and analysis. Additionally, the study may be subject to selection bias, as patients were not randomized to different embolizing particle size groups and it was conducted at a single center. Factors influencing the choice of particle size may have confounded the observed outcomes. The follow-up period in our study was relatively short-term, with outcomes assessed at 6 months and 1 year after the procedure. Moreover, the inclusion of patients treated with a range of embolizing particle sizes introduces variability in outcomes.

Lastly, while our study analyzed outcomes based on embolizing particle size, it did not directly compare the efficacy and safety of different particle sizes to the small sample size.

## 5. Conclusions

In conclusion, our study underscores the significance of prostatic artery embolization (PAE) as a viable treatment option for Benign Prostatic Hyperplasia (BPH). While achieving technical success and favorable outcomes in catheter removal, our findings highlight the importance of individualizing treatment approaches based on embolizing particle size. The results of our study emphasise that small particles are very effective in reducing prostate volume and thus BPH-related LUTS with few side effects. However, the study's limitations, including sample size constraints and retrospective design, necessitate cautious interpretation of the results. Moving forward, further research efforts should prioritize larger, prospective studies to validate our findings and optimize patient care in BPH management. Despite these limitations, our study adds valuable insights to the existing literature, reaffirming PAE's role as a safe and effective minimally invasive intervention for patients with BPH.

**Author Contributions:** Conceptualization, G.X.; Data curation, L.V.S., A.V. and A.E.C.; Formal analysis, L.V.S., A.V. and A.E.C.; Funding acquisition, G.X. and F.D.G.; Investigation, L.V.S. and A.V.; Project administration, G.X.; Supervision, G.X., F.D.G., A.M.I. and G.C.; Validation, G.X., L.V.S., A.V. and F.D.G.; Visualization, L.V.S., A.V., A.E.C., V.A., A.R., A.A.I., A.I., P.N., A.M.I. and G.C.; Writing—original draft, L.V.S. and A.V.; Writing—review and editing, G.X., L.V.S. and A.V. All authors have read and agreed to the published version of the manuscript.

**Funding:** This research received no external funding.

**Institutional Review Board Statement:** Not applicable.

**Informed Consent Statement:** Informed consent was obtained from all subjects involved in the study.

**Data Availability Statement:** All data are available.

**Conflicts of Interest:** The authors declare no conflicts of interest.

## References

1. Sayegh, N.; Gross, K. Benign prostatic hyperplasia: A global challenge of the ageing population. *Lancet Healthy Longev.* **2022**, *3*, e725–e726. [CrossRef] [PubMed]
2. Parsons, J.K. Benign Prostatic Hyperplasia and Male Lower Urinary Tract Symptoms: Epidemiology and Risk Factors. *Curr. Bladder Dysfunct. Rep.* **2010**, *5*, 212–218. [CrossRef] [PubMed]
3. Rastrelli, G.; Vignozzi, L.; Corona, G.; Maggi, M. Testosterone and Benign Prostatic Hyperplasia. *Sex. Med. Rev.* **2019**, *7*, 259–271. [CrossRef] [PubMed]
4. Xia, B.W.; Zhao, S.C.; Chen, Z.P.; Chen, C.; Liu, T.S.; Yang, F.; Yan, Y. Relationship between serum total testosterone and prostate volume in aging men. *Sci. Rep.* **2021**, *11*, 14122. [CrossRef] [PubMed]
5. Parsons, J.K.; Bergstrom, J.; Silberstein, J.; Barrett-Connor, E. Prevalence and characteristics of lower urinary tract symptoms in men aged > or = 80 years. *Urology* **2008**, *72*, 318–321. [CrossRef] [PubMed]
6. Chalise, P.R.; Agrawal, C.S. Change in urinary symptoms and quality of life in men with benign prostatic hyperplasia after transurethral resection of prostate. *Nepal Med. Coll. J.* **2007**, *9*, 255–258. [PubMed]
7. Jacobsen, S.J.; Jacobson, D.J.; Girman, C.J.; Roberts, R.O.; Rhodes, T.; Guess, H.A.; Lieber, M.M. Natural history of prostatism: Risk factors for acute urinary retention. *J. Urol.* **1997**, *158*, 481–487. [CrossRef] [PubMed]
8. Zattoni, F.; Ficarra, V.; Novara, G. Risk stratification for benign prostatic hyperplasia. *Urologia* **2017**, *84*, 153–157. [CrossRef] [PubMed]
9. Roehrborn, C.G. The epidemiology of acute urinary retention in benign prostatic hyperplasia. *Rev. Urol.* **2001**, *3*, 187–192.
10. Muruganandham, K.; Dubey, D.; Kapoor, R. Acute urinary retention in benign prostatic hyperplasia: Risk factors and current management. *Indian J. Urol.* **2007**, *23*, 347–353. [CrossRef]
11. Gravas, S.; Gacci, M.; Gratzke, C.; Herrmann, T.R.; Karavitakis, M.; Kyriazis, I.; Malde, S.; Mamoulakis, C.; Rieken, M.; Sakalis, V.I.; et al. Summary Paper on the 2023 European Association of Urology Guidelines on the Management of Non-neurogenic Male Lower Urinary Tract Symptoms. *Eur. Urol.* **2023**, *84*, 207–222. [CrossRef] [PubMed]

12. Roehrborn, C.G.; Siami, P.; Barkin, J.; Damião, R.; Major-Walker, K.; Nandy, I.; Morrill, B.B.; Gagnier, R.P.; Montorsi, F.; CombAT Study Group. The effects of combination therapy with dutasteride and tamsulosin on clinical outcomes in men with symptomatic benign prostatic hyperplasia: 4-year results from the CombAT study. *Eur. Urol.* **2010**, *57*, 123–131. [CrossRef] [PubMed]
13. Lerner, L.B.; McVary, K.T.; Barry, M.J.; Bixler, B.R.; Dahm, P.; Das, A.K.; Gandhi, M.C.; Kaplan, S.A.; Kohler, T.S.; Martin, L.; et al. Management of Lower Urinary Tract Symptoms Attributed to Benign Prostatic Hyperplasia: AUA GUIDELINE PART II-Surgical Evaluation and Treatment. *J. Urol.* **2021**, *206*, 818–826. [CrossRef] [PubMed]
14. Oelke, M.; Bachmann, A.; Descazeaud, A.; Emberton, M.; Gravas, S.; Michel, M.C.; N'dow, J.; Nordling, J.; de la Rosette, J.J. EAU guidelines on the treatment and follow-up of non-neurogenic male lower urinary tract symptoms including benign prostatic obstruction. *Eur. Urol.* **2013**, *64*, 118–140. [CrossRef] [PubMed]
15. Sandhu, J.S.; Bixler, B.R.; Dahm, P.; Goueli, R.; Kirkby, E.; Stoffel, J.T.; Wilt, T.J. Management of Lower Urinary Tract Symptoms Attributed to Benign Prostatic Hyperplasia (BPH): AUA Guideline Amendment 2023. *J. Urol.* **2024**, *211*, 11–19. [CrossRef]
16. Sciacqua, L.V.; Vanzulli, A.; Di Meo, R.; Pellegrino, G.; Lavorato, R.; Vitale, G.; Carrafiello, G. Minimally Invasive Treatment in Benign Prostatic Hyperplasia (BPH). *Technol. Cancer Res. Treat.* **2023**, *22*, 15330338231155000. [CrossRef] [PubMed]
17. Cornu, J.N.; Ahyai, S.; Bachmann, A.; de la Rosette, J.; Gilling, P.; Gratzke, C.; McVary, K.; Novara, G.; Woo, H.; Madersbacher, S. A Systematic Review and Meta-analysis of Functional Outcomes and Complications Following Transurethral Procedures for Lower Urinary Tract Symptoms Resulting from Benign Prostatic Obstruction: An Update. *Eur. Urol.* **2015**, *67*, 1066–1096. [CrossRef]
18. Iqbal, J.; Mashkoor, Y.; Nadeem, A.; Tah, S.; Sharifa, M.; Ghani, S.; Thugu, T.R.; Patel, H.; Bonner-Reid, F.T.; Shrestha, J.; et al. Shifting Trends in Prostate Treatment: A Systematic Review Comparing Transurethral Resection of the Prostate and Holmium Laser Enucleation of the Prostate. *Cureus* **2023**, *15*, e46173. [CrossRef] [PubMed]
19. Hahn, R.G. The transurethral resection syndrome. *Acta Anaesthesiol. Scand.* **1991**, *35*, 557–567. [CrossRef]
20. Demirel, I.; Ozer, A.B.; Bayar, M.K.; Erhan, O.L. TURP syndrome and severe hyponatremia under general anaesthesia. *BMJ Case Rep.* **2012**, *2012*, bcr-2012. [CrossRef]
21. Rassweiler, J.; Teber, D.; Kuntz, R.; Hofmann, R. Complications of transurethral resection of the prostate (TURP)--incidence, management, and prevention. *Eur. Urol.* **2006**, *50*, 969–979; discussion 980. [CrossRef] [PubMed]
22. Augestad, K.M.; Berntsen, G.; Lassen, K.; Bellika, J.G.; Wootton, R.; Lindsetmo, R.O.; Study Group of Research Quality in Medical Informatics and Decision Support (SQUID). Standards for reporting randomized controlled trials in medical informatics: A systematic review of CONSORT adherence in RCTs on clinical decision support. *J. Am. Med. Inform. Assoc.* **2012**, *19*, 13–21. [CrossRef] [PubMed]
23. Tan, A.H.H.; Gilling, P.J.; Kennett, K.M.; Frampton, C.; Westenberg, A.M.; Fraundorfer, M.R. A randomized trial comparing holmium laser enucleation of the prostate with transurethral resection of the prostate for the treatment of bladder outlet obstruction secondary to benign prostatic hyperplasia in large glands (40 to 200 grams). *J. Urol.* **2003**, *170 Pt 1*, 1270–1274. [CrossRef] [PubMed]
24. Khater, U.; Smith, N.A.; Katz, J.E.; Bhat, A.; Banerjee, I.; Shah, R.H.; Shah, H.N. Does prior transurethral resection of prostate have a negative impact on the outcome of holmium laser enucleation of prostate? Results from a prospective comparative study. *Urol. Ann.* **2022**, *14*, 118–124. [CrossRef] [PubMed]
25. Jhanwar, A.; Sinha, R.J.; Bansal, A.; Prakash, G.; Singh, K.; Singh, V. Outcomes of transurethral resection and holmium laser enucleation in more than 60 g of prostate: A prospective randomized study. *Urol. Ann.* **2017**, *9*, 45–50. [CrossRef] [PubMed]
26. Fayad, A.S.; Elsheikh, M.G.; Zakaria, T.; Elfottoh, H.A.; Alsergany, R.; Elshenoufy, A.; Elghamarawy, H. Holmium Laser Enucleation of the Prostate Versus Bipolar Resection of the Prostate: A Prospective Randomized Study. 'Pros and Cons'. *Urology* **2015**, *86*, 1037–1041. [CrossRef] [PubMed]
27. Chen, F.; Chen, Y.; Zou, Y.; Wang, Y.; Wu, X.; Chen, M. Comparison of holmium laser enucleation and transurethral resection of prostate in benign prostatic hyperplasia: A systematic review and meta-analysis. *J. Int. Med. Res.* **2023**, *51*, 3000605231190763. [CrossRef] [PubMed]
28. Tzeng, M.; Basourakos, S.P.; Lewicki, P.J.; Hu, J.C.; Lee, R.K. New Endoscopic In-office Surgical Therapies for Benign Prostatic Hyperplasia: A Systematic Review. *Eur. Urol. Focus* **2022**, *8*, 522–531. [CrossRef]
29. Yang, J.; Wu, W.; Amier, Y.; Li, X.; Wan, W.; Liu, C.; Zhang, Y.; Yu, X. Efficacy and safety of Water Vapor Thermal Therapy in the treatment of benign prostate hyperplasia: A systematic review and single-arm Meta-analysis. *BMC Urol.* **2023**, *23*, 72. [CrossRef]
30. Warli, S.M.; Ikram, M.F.; Sarumpaet, R.G.; Tala, Z.Z.; Putrantyo, I.I. The efficacy and safety of prostatic urethral lift as a minimally invasive therapeutic modality to treat lower urinary tract symptoms while maintaining sexual function in patients with benign prostatic hyperplasia: A systematic review and meta-analysis of randomized controlled trials. *Arch. Ital. Urol. Androl.* **2024**, *96*, 12066. [CrossRef]
31. Cornu, J.N.; Zantek, P.; Burtt, G.; Martin, C.; Martin, A.; Springate, C.; Chughtai, B. Minimally Invasive Treatments for Benign Prostatic Obstruction: A Systematic Review and Network Meta-analysis. *Eur. Urol.* **2023**, *83*, 534–547. [CrossRef] [PubMed]
32. Williams, D.R.A. *Minimally-Invasive Treatments for Lower Urinary Tract Symptoms in People with Benign Prostatic Hyperplasia: A Review of Clinical Effectiveness*; Canadian Agency for Drugs and Technologies in Health: Ottawa, ON, Canada, 2021.
33. Braun, M.; Mathers, M.; Bondarenko, B.; Engelmann, U. Treatment of benign prostatic hyperplasia through transurethral needle ablation (TUNA). Review of the literature and six years of clinical experience. *Urol. Int.* **2004**, *72*, 32–39. [CrossRef] [PubMed]

34. Law, Y.X.T.; Chen, W.J.K.; Shen, L.; Chua, W.J. Is transurethral needle ablation of prostate out of fashion? Outcomes of single session office-based transurethral needle ablation of prostate in patients with symptomatic benign prostatic hyperplasia. *Investig. Clin. Urol.* **2019**, *60*, 351–358. [CrossRef] [PubMed]
35. Walmsley, K.; Kaplan, S.A. Transurethral microwave thermotherapy for benign prostate hyperplasia: Separating truth from marketing hype. *J. Urol.* **2004**, *172 Pt 1*, 1249–1255. [CrossRef]
36. Franco, J.V.A.; Garegnani, L.; Liquitay, C.M.E.; Borofsky, M.; Dahm, P. Transurethral Microwave Thermotherapy for Benign Prostatic Hyperplasia: An Updated Cochrane Review. *World J. Mens. Health* **2022**, *40*, 127–138. [CrossRef] [PubMed]
37. Ghanouni, P.; Gill, H.; Kaye, E.; Pauly, K.B.; Daniel, B. MR imaging-guided cryoablation for the treatment of benign prostatic hyperplasia. *J. Vasc. Interv. Radiol.* **2011**, *22*, 1427–1430. [CrossRef] [PubMed]
38. Wang, A.; Wang, D.; Tong, W. Cryosurgical ablation for aged patients with severe benign prostate hyperplasia: A report of 21 cases. *Zhonghua Nan Ke Xue = Natl. J. Androl.* **2007**, *13*, 421–423.
39. McWilliams, J.P.; Kuo, M.D.; Rose, S.C.; Bagla, S.; Caplin, D.M.; Cohen, E.I.; Faintuch, S.; Spies, J.B.; Saad, W.E.; Nikolic, B. Society of Interventional Radiology Position Statement: Prostate Artery Embolization for Treatment of Benign Disease of the Prostate. *J. Vasc. Interv. Radiol.* **2014**, *25*, 1349–1351. [CrossRef] [PubMed]
40. Qamhawi, Z.; Little, M.W. The State of Evidence in Prostate Artery Embolization. *Semin. Intervent. Radiol.* **2022**, *39*, 571–576. [CrossRef]
41. Goyal, P.; Salem, R.; Mouli, S.K. Controversies in Prostate Artery Embolization: Future Best Practice. *Semin. Intervent. Radiol.* **2022**, *39*, 562–570. [CrossRef]
42. Carnevale, F.C.; Moreira, A.M.; de Assis, A.M.; Antunes, A.A.; Cristina de Paula Rodrigues, V.; Srougi, M.; Cerri, G.G. Prostatic Artery Embolization for the Treatment of Lower Urinary Tract Symptoms Due to Benign Prostatic Hyperplasia: 10 Years' Experience. *Radiology* **2020**, *296*, 444–451. [CrossRef]
43. Cizman, Z.; Isaacson, A.; Burke, C. Short- to Midterm Safety and Efficacy of Prostatic Artery Embolization: A Systematic Review. *J. Vasc. Interv. Radiol.* **2016**, *27*, 1487–1493.e1. [CrossRef]
44. DeMeritt, J.S.; Elmasri, F.F.; Esposito, M.P.; Rosenberg, G.S. Relief of benign prostatic hyperplasia-related bladder outlet obstruction after transarterial polyvinyl alcohol prostate embolization. *J. Vasc. Interv. Radiol.* **2000**, *11*, 767–770. [CrossRef]
45. Bilhim, T. Prostatic Artery Embolization: An Update. *Korean J. Radiol.* **2023**, *24*, 313–323. [CrossRef]
46. Bilhim, T.; Costa, N.V.; Torres, D.; Pinheiro, L.C.; Spaepen, E. Long-Term Outcome of Prostatic Artery Embolization for Patients with Benign Prostatic Hyperplasia: Single-Centre Retrospective Study in 1072 Patients Over a 10-Year Period. *Cardiovasc. Intervent. Radiol.* **2022**, *45*, 1324–1336. [CrossRef]
47. Gonçalves, O.M.; Carnevale, F.C.; Moreira, A.M.; Antunes, A.A.; Rodrigues, V.C.; Srougi, M. Comparative Study Using 100-300 Versus 300-500 μm Microspheres for Symptomatic Patients Due to Enlarged-BPH Prostates. *Cardiovasc. Intervent. Radiol.* **2016**, *39*, 1372–1378. [CrossRef] [PubMed]
48. Torres, D.; Costa, N.V.; Pisco, J.; Pinheiro, L.C.; Oliveira, A.G.; Bilhim, T. Prostatic Artery Embolization for Benign Prostatic Hyperplasia: Prospective Randomized Trial of 100-300 μm versus 300-500 μm versus 100- to 300-μm + 300- to 500-μm Embospheres. *J. Vasc. Interv. Radiol.* **2019**, *30*, 638–644. [CrossRef] [PubMed]
49. Bilhim, T.; Pisco, J.; Pinheiro, L.C.; Tinto, H.R.; Fernandes, L.; Pereira, J.A.; Duarte, M.; Oliveira, A.G. Does polyvinyl alcohol particle size change the outcome of prostatic arterial embolization for benign prostatic hyperplasia? Results from a single-center randomized prospective study. *J. Vasc. Interv. Radiol.* **2013**, *24*, 1595–1602.e1. [CrossRef] [PubMed]
50. Baerlocher, M.O.; Nikolic, B.; Sze, D.Y. Adverse Event Classification: Clarification and Validation of the Society of Interventional Radiology Specialty-Specific System. *J. Vasc. Interv. Radiol.* **2023**, *34*, S1051-0443. [CrossRef]
51. Khalilzadeh, O.; Baerlocher, M.O.; Shyn, P.B.; Connolly, B.L.; Devane, A.M.; Morris, C.S.; Cohen, A.M.; Midia, M.; Thornton, R.H.; Gross, K.; et al. Proposal of a New Adverse Event Classification by the Society of Interventional Radiology Standards of Practice Committee. *J. Vasc. Interv. Radiol.* **2017**, *28*, 1432–1437.e3. [CrossRef]
52. Bhatia, S.; Sinha, V.K.; Kava, B.R.; Gomez, C.; Harward, S.; Punnen, S.; Kably, I.; Miller, J.; Parekh, D.J. Efficacy of Prostatic Artery Embolization for Catheter-Dependent Patients with Large Prostate Sizes and High Comorbidity Scores. *J. Vasc. Interv. Radiol.* **2018**, *29*, 78–84.e1. [CrossRef] [PubMed]
53. Patel, S.R.; Lowrey, K.A.; Johny, A.; Smith, C.P. Improvement in International Prostate Symptom Score after prostatic urethral lifts is dependent on prostatic volume. *Can. J. Urol.* **2023**, *30*, 11619–11623. [PubMed]
54. Wolters, M.; Krastel, M.; Winkler, T.; Idais, H.; Mazdak, M.; Tezval, H.; Kuczyk, M.A.; von Klot, C.J. Real-world experience of water vapour therapy (Rezum) in patients with benign prostatic enlargement: A retrospective single-center study. *Prostate Cancer Prostatic Dis* **2024**. [CrossRef] [PubMed]
55. McVary, K.T.; Miller, L.E.; Bhattacharyya, S.; DeRouen, K.; Turner, E.; Zantek, P.; Abdel Rassoul, M.; Miyauchi, T.; Alzahrani, T.M.; Kohler, T. Water Vapor Thermal Therapy in Men With Prostate Volume ≥80 cm (3): A Systematic Review and Meta-Analysis. *Urology* **2024**, *184*, 244–250. [CrossRef] [PubMed]
56. Zell, M.A.; Abdul-Muhsin, H.; Navaratnam, A.; Cumsky, J.; Girardo, M.; Cornella, J.; Nevo, A.; Cheney, S.; Humphreys, M.R. Holmium laser enucleation of the prostate for very large benign prostatic hyperplasia (≥ 200 cc). *World J. Urol.* **2021**, *39*, 129–134. [CrossRef] [PubMed]

57. Veyg, D.; Mohanka, R.; Rumball, I.P.; Liang, R.; Garcia-Reyes, K.; Bishay, V.; Fischman, A.M. Comparison of 24-Month Clinical Outcomes after Prostatic Artery Embolization in Prostate Glands Larger versus Smaller than 80 mL: A Systematic Review. *J. Vasc. Interv. Radiol.* **2023**, *34*, 578–584.e1. [CrossRef]
58. Wang, M.Q.; Zhang, J.L.; Xin, H.N.; Yuan, K.; Yan, J.; Wang, Y.; Zhang, G.D.; Fu, J.X. Comparison of Clinical Outcomes of Prostatic Artery Embolization with 50-µm Plus 100-µm Polyvinyl Alcohol (PVA) Particles versus 100-µm PVA Particles Alone: A Prospective Randomized Trial. *J. Vasc. Interv. Radiol.* **2018**, *29*, 1694–1702. [CrossRef]

Journal of Personalized Medicine

MDPI

*Article*

# The Deterioration of Sarcopenia Post-Transarterial Radioembolization with Holmium-166 Serves as a Predictor for Disease Progression at 3 Months in Patients with Advanced Hepatocellular Carcinoma: A Pilot Study

**Claudio Trobiani [1], Nicolò Ubaldi [2,*], Leonardo Teodoli [1], Marcello Andrea Tipaldi [2], Federico Cappelli [1], Sara Ungania [3] and Giulio Vallati [1]**

1 Interventional Radiology Unit, "IRCCS Istituto Nazionale Tumori Regina Elena", 00144 Rome, Italy; claudio.trobiani@ifo.it (C.T.); leonardo.teodoli@ifo.it (L.T.); federico.cappelli@ifo.it (F.C.); giulio.vallati@ifo.it (G.V.)

2 Department of Medical Surgical Sciences and Translational Medicine, Sapienza-University of Rome, Radiology Unit–Sant'Andrea Hospital, 1035 Via Di Grottarossa, 00189 Rome, Italy; tipaldi.andrea@gmail.com

3 Medical Physics Department, "IRCCS Istituto Nazionale Tumori Regina Elena", 00144 Rome, Italy; sara.ungania@ifo.it

* Correspondence: ubaldi.nicolo@gmail.com

**Abstract:** Purpose: The aim of this pilot study is to explore the relationship between changes in sarcopenia before and after one to three months of Transarterial Radioembolization (TARE) treatment with Holmium-166 (166Ho) and its effect on the rate of local response. Our primary objective is to assess whether the worsening of sarcopenia can function as an early indicator of a subgroup of patients at increased risk of disease progression in cases of hepatocellular carcinoma (HCC). Methods: A single-center retrospective analysis was performed on 25 patients with HCC who underwent 166Ho-TARE. Sarcopenia status was defined according to the measurement of the psoas muscle index (PMI) at baseline, one month, and three months after TARE. Radiological response according to mRECIST criteria was assessed and patients were grouped into responders and non-responders. The loco-regional response rate was evaluated for all patients before and after treatment, and was compared with sarcopenia status to identify any potential correlation. Results: A total of 20 patients were analyzed. According to the sarcopenia status at 1 month and 3 months, two groups were defined as follows: patients in which the deltaPMI was stable or increased (No-Sarcopenia group; $n = 12$) vs. patients in which the deltaPMI decreased (Sarcopenia group; $n = 8$). Three months after TARE, a significant difference in sarcopenia status was noted ($p = 0.041$) between the responders and non-responders, with the non-responder group showing a decrease in the sarcopenia values with a median deltaPMI of −0.57, compared to a median deltaPMI of 0.12 in the responder group. Therefore, deltaPMI measured three months post-TARE can be considered as a predictive biomarker for the local response rate ($p = 0.028$). Lastly, a minor deltaPMI variation (>−0.293) was found to be indicative of positive treatment outcomes ($p = 0.0001$). Conclusion: The decline in sarcopenia three months post-TARE with Holmium-166 is a reliable predictor of worse loco-regional response rate, as evaluated radiologically, in patients with HCC. Sarcopenia measurement has the potential to be a valuable assessment tool in the management of HCC patients undergoing TARE. However, further prospective and randomized studies involving larger cohorts are necessary to confirm and validate these findings.

**Keywords:** TARE; sarcopenia; HCC; interventional oncology; liver; Holmium-166

## 1. Introduction

Primary liver cancer was diagnosed in roughly 800,000 patients worldwide in 2022, accounting for more than 700,000 deaths annually [1]. Transarterial Radioembolization

(TARE) is a minimally invasive treatment that combines low-volume arterial embolization with internal radiation therapy. It is commonly used for unresectable hepatocellular carcinoma (HCC) and is generally regarded as safe and effective, showing improvements in overall survival compared to conventional treatments [2]. Initially developed as a palliative treatment in the 1960s [3], by late 2022, TARE had been incorporated into the early-stage section (i.e., BCLC 0-A) of the Barcelona Clinic Liver Cancer algorithm, particularly in cases where other HCC treatments have failed or are not feasible [4]. A recent phase II randomized trial (TRACE) comparing TARE to transarterial chemoembolization (TACE) in patients with early- or intermediate-stage HCC revealed that TARE provided superior tumor control and overall survival outcomes [5]. Compared to TACE, TARE is associated with lower toxicity to healthy liver tissue and reduced static embolization effects, potentially resulting in less hepatocyte damage and better tolerability, particularly in patients with portal vein thrombosis [6,7]. Patient selection for TARE involves evaluation by a multidisciplinary oncology team, typically considering individuals with a life expectancy of more than three months, bilirubin levels below 2 mg/dL, albumin levels above 3 g/dL, and an Eastern Cooperative Oncology Group status of 2 or lower [8].

Various radioactive isotopes are employed for Transarterial Radioembolization (TARE), with Yttrium-90 (90Y) being the most commonly utilized and the longest established option, although Holmium-166 (166Ho) microspheres have recently become available as an alternative. 166Ho microspheres received a CE mark under the commercial name of QuiremSpheres™ (Quirem BV, Deventer, The Netherlands) in 2015. The basis of 166Ho is Poly-L-lactic acid, offering distinct advantages over Yttrium-90. It possesses both high-energy beta emission for the treatment process and lower gamma emission for scoping, with the latter assessed using SPECT imaging. Additionally, due to its paramagnetic properties, MRI facilitates convenient assessment of tumor dose distribution and quantification [9,10]. Typically, 166Ho is loaded into either resin or glass microspheres, with resin being more readily available but having lower density [8]. Holmium has a relatively medium–short half-life of 26.8 h, resulting in a high dose rate over a brief period. This allows for the evaluation of treatment response through CT, FDG-PET, or MRI at shorter intervals compared to 90Y, typically <6 months in our clinical practice. This innovative treatment has seen potential benefits in improving intrahepatic distribution prediction compared with current standard treatment [9]. Up to now, Holmium microspheres have only been recently used in clinical practice; specifically, less than 10 clinical trials have been carried out [9], of which the most recent were the HEPAR Primary study, which assessed HCC [11], and the HORA EST clinical trial, which assessed early HCC [12], evaluating the efficacy and toxicity profiles.

Several prognostic staging systems have been developed for HCC; however, they often overlook patients' performance status [13]. Sarcopenia, defined as the "progressive loss of muscle mass and strength with a risk of adverse outcomes such as disability, poor quality of life, and death" [12], manifests relatively early in HCC and can independently negatively predict HCC-related mortality in patients undergoing loco-regional treatment [13–15]. Indeed, sarcopenia has been associated with poor treatment response in HCC [16] and has recently been identified as a predictor of progressive disease in HCC treated with TARE-90Y [15]. Given that sarcopenia could be used to assess the overall response to loco-regional HCC treatment [15,17,18], it is crucial to identify patients with worsening sarcopenia, as they might benefit from early loco-regional re-treatment and nutritional support to restore muscle mass and strength. To the best of our knowledge, there have been no other studies evaluating a treatment response predictor, such as sarcopenia status, following TARE-166Ho for HCC.

The aim of this preliminary study is to assess whether there is a potential relationship between changes in sarcopenia before and after one–three months of TARE-166Ho treatment and the rate of local response it induces, and thus to determine if the deterioration of sarcopenia worsening can serve as an early identifier of a subgroup of patients who are at a high risk of disease progression.

## 2. Materials and Methods

### 2.1. Patients

A retrospective investigation was conducted on patients with BCLC-B large monofocal or multifocal HCC who underwent TARE-166Ho in the period 2022–2023. The sarcopenia status was defined according to the measurement of the psoas muscle index (PMI), as described later, at baseline, one month, and three months after TARE. The population was divided into two groups according to sarcopenia status: patients in which the deltaPMI was stable or increased (No-Sarcopenia group) and patients in which the deltaPMI decreased (Sarcopenia group). The radiological response, according to mRECIST criteria, was assessed one and three months subsequent to the procedure and patients were grouped into responders and non-responders. Throughout the follow-up period, patients did not modify their exercise and nutrition habits from baseline. All methods or experimental protocols were approved by the local institutional review board and were carried out in accordance with the relevant guidelines of the Declaration of Helsinki. Informed consent was collected from all participants.

### 2.2. Sarcopenia Measurement

Sarcopenia manifests as a syndrome marked by gradual and widespread decline in skeletal muscle mass and strength, closely associated with physical impairment, diminished quality of life, and mortality [19]. The assessment of sarcopenia status was determined by measuring the PMI before and after treatment. Sarcopenia was confirmed in patients with reduced PMI after treatment. The PMI was calculated using the following formula: PMI [mm/m$^2$]: [(minor diameter of left psoas + major diameter of left psoas + minor diameter of right psoas + major diameter of right psoas)/4]/height in m$^2$ [20]. All the psoas measurements were performed at the level of L3-L4 (Figures 1 and 2) on multiphasic CT scans performed in the same center having all identical slice thickness.

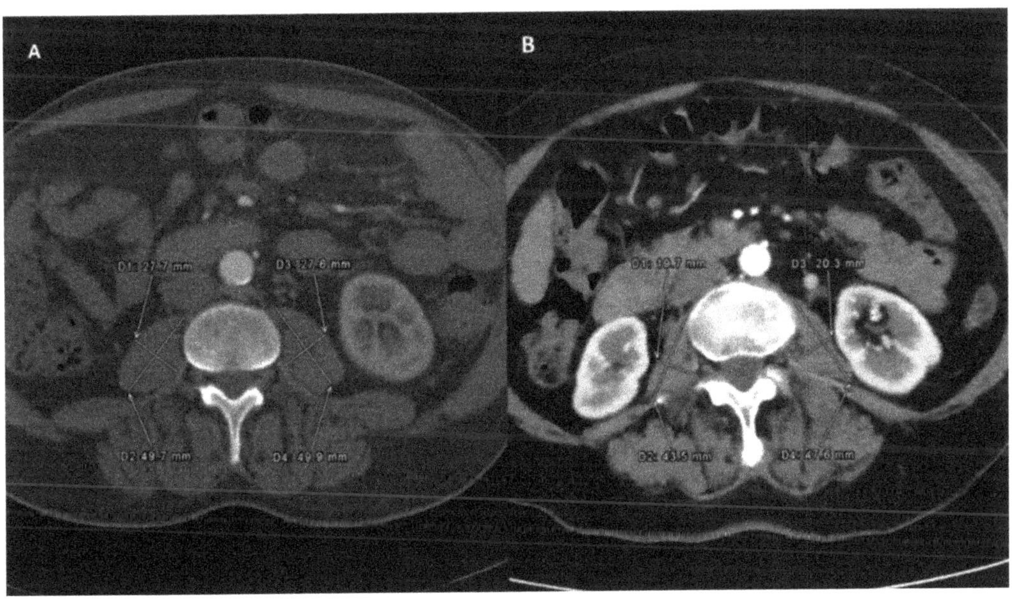


**Figure 1.** Sarcopenia status measured before TARE in the Sarcopenia group (**A**) and the No-Sarcopenia group (**B**).

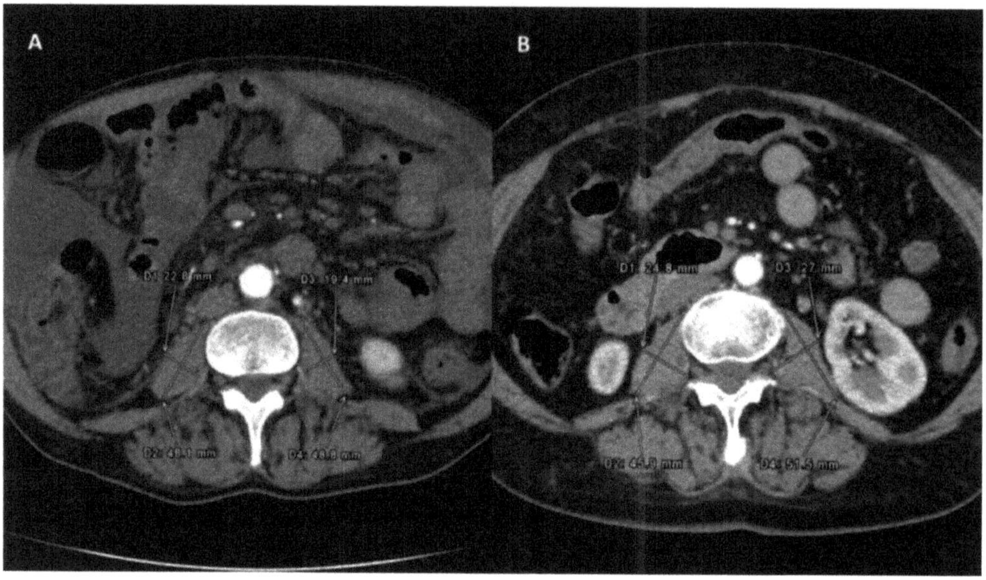


**Figure 2.** Sarcopenia status measured after TARE in the Sarcopenia group (**A**) and the No-Sarcopenia group (**B**).

## 2.3. TARE

All procedures were carried out by experienced interventional radiologists with more than five years of experience. For the treatment, 80–170 MBq 166mHo-loaded scout microspheres were administered slowly through a 2.7-F micro-catheter (Progreat; Terumo Europe NV, Leuven, Belgium) placed in the pathological feeder artery. The distribution of the drug was assessed using SPECT imaging. Post-therapy SPECT/CT scans (Symbia IntevoTM system; Siemens, Erlangen, Germany) were performed between 1 and 20 h after SIRT to evaluate the distribution of the microspheres thanks to 2D and 3D dosimetry maps.

Firstly, the accuracy and intensity of the 166Ho microspheres' activity distribution were evaluated by analyzing the 2D activity intensity peak (Pixel Value) of the signal along a line crossing the treated area. A higher peak indicated a more intense signal within the targeted area.

Later, the 3D effective dose in Gy distributed to the lesion and liver parenchyma per unit cumulated activity (GBq), was calculated according to the activity distribution obtained from SPECT/CT imaging, utilizing a MIM 6.1.7 workstation (MIM Software Inc., Cleveland, OH, USA). For each patient, the mean absorbed dose (<D>) in Gy for the normal liver and tumor were compared with the expected values (<D> to tumor > 100 Gy, <D> to normal liver < 40 Gy) to assess the treatment efficacy.

## 2.4. Statistical Analysis

The Mann–Whitney U test was used for evaluating the deltaPMI according to treatment response at 1 and 3 months after TARE. The PMI at the time of TARE was compared with the PMI measurements at one and three months after TARE. The deltaPMI measurements between the first PMI measurement and the controls at one and three months were evaluated. Variables with a $p < 0.05$ were considered statistically significant.

The accuracy of the different sarcopenia measurements performed over time was assessed through c-statistics analysis, with the intent to evaluate their ability to predict progressive disease after TARE. Areas under the curve (AUCs) and 95% CI were reported. Fisher's exact test was used for comparisons of categorical variables.

## 3. Results

Between 2022 and 2023, a total of 25 patients with BCLC-B HCC underwent TARE-166Ho. Five patients were excluded from the study due to drop-out and the absence of post-treatment follow-up CT scans. The patients' demographics and clinical features did not differ between the two sarcopenia groups and are depicted in Table 1. Additionally, tumor characteristics at the time of TARE were similar between the two groups, in terms of maximum diameter of target nodule ($p$ = 0.60), number of lesions ($p$ = 0.43), and bilobar involvement of the disease ($p$ = 0.84). Also, PMI at baseline was not significant between the two groups ($p$ = 0.79). Lastly, the HCC biological markers, such as alpha-fetoprotein (AFP) and protein induced by vitamin K absence (PIVKA), were similar between the two groups.

**Table 1.** Patient population demographics and clinical characteristics.

| Variable | No-Sarcopenia Group ($n$ = 12) | Sarcopenia Group ($n$ = 8) | $p$ |
|---|---|---|---|
| | Median (IQR) or $n$ (%) | | |
| Age (years) | 63 (58–67) | 63 (57–70) | 0.44 |
| Male sex | 7 (58.3) | 5 (62.5) | 0.78 |
| Height (cm) | 170 (162–180) | 174 (165–180) | 0.32 |
| Ascites (any grade) | 4 (33.3) | 2 (25) | 0.78 |
| Moderate | 1 (8.3) | 1 (12.5) | |
| Maximum size of treated lesion (mm) | 45 (33–71) | 50 (35–78) | 0.60 |
| Number of lesions | 2 (1–4) | 3 (2–4) | 0.43 |
| Bilobar involvement | 7 (58.3) | 4 (50) | 0.84 |
| Liver parenchyma involved > 50% | 3 (25) | 2 (25) | 1.00 |
| Bilobar TARE treatment | 7 (58.3) | 4 (50) | 0.67 |
| AFP measure (ng/mL) pre-procedural | 58 (19–235) | 69 (26–210) | 0.85 |
| PIVKA measure (AU/mL) pre-procedural | 155 (93–436) | 172 (44–445) | 0.89 |
| PMI (mm/m$^2$) at baseline | 12 (6–16) | 12 (8–13) | 0.79 |

Abbreviations: $n$, number; IQR, interquartile ranges.

Furthermore, no statistical differences were observed between the two groups in terms of liver function features or disease burden. Additionally, no disparities were found between the groups regarding administered dose activity: the mean activity administered in Gigabequerels (GBq) was 4.5 (3.60–8.82) in the Sarcopenia group and 5.1 (2.62–9.08) in the No-Sarcopenia group. The technical success of TARE was 100%, with the administration of 166Ho microspheres within the tumor-feeding artery reached in all cases. No post-procedural complications were reported in either group.

Dose activity metrics in TARE, in terms of activity intensity peak and mean absorbed dose to the tumor and to the liver, were calculated and compared between the two sarcopenia groups, as shown in Table 2. Regarding the efficacy of TARE, it demonstrated a favorable dosimetrical profile in both 2D and 3D analysis. In terms of 2D evaluation, no statistical differences were found between the groups in terms of activity intensity peak calculated in grayscale (903.8 ± 110.1 in the Sarcopenia group vs. 998.6 ± 94.9 in the No-Sarcopenia group, $p$ = 0.21). For 3D dose analysis (expressed as absorbed dose in Gy), the mean absorbed dose to normal liver (<Dnliver>) was <40 Gy for both groups, with no significant differences observed (26.0 ± 5.2 Gy in the Sarcopenia group vs. 29.5 ± 9.8 Gy in the No-Sarcopenia group, $p$ = 0.50).

Similarly, the mean absorbed dose to the tumor (<Dtumor>) was calculated for all patients, with no statistical differences between the groups (154.2 ± 56.7 in the Sarcopenia group vs. 162.7 ± 47.8 in the No-Sarcopenia group, $p$ = 0.13). Additionally, the mean absorbed dose to normal liver (<Dnliver>) remained <40 Gy for both groups, with no significant differences (26.0 ± 5.2 Gy vs. 29.5 ± 9.8 Gy, $p$ = 0.50).

**Table 2.** Comparison of dose activity metrics in TARE between Sarcopenia and No-Sarcopenia groups.

| | Sarcopenia Group n = 8 | No-Sarcopenia Group n = 12 | $p$ |
|---|---|---|---|
| Activity intensity peak (Grayscale) | 903.8 ± 110.1 | 998.6 ± 94.9 | 0.21 |
| <Dtumor> (Gy) | 154.2 ± 56.7 | 162.7 ± 47.8 | 0.13 |
| <Dnliver> (Gy) | 26.0 ± 5.2 | 29.5 ± 9.8 | 0.40 |

According to the sarcopenia status, measured as the deltaPMI before and after treatment at 1 month and 3 months, two groups were defined as follows: patients in which the deltaPMI was stable or increased (No-Sarcopenia group; $n = 12$) vs. patients in which the deltaPMI decreased (Sarcopenia group; $n = 8$).

The radiological response rate was evaluated for all patients one month and three months after the TARE procedure, and patients were grouped as follows: those with standard and progressive disease were added to the non-responder group, and those with complete response or partial response were added to the responder group.

The local response rate was compared with the sarcopenia status at 1 and 3 months.

At 1 month, no statistically significant difference ($p = 0.229$) was observed in terms of sarcopenia status, with a median deltaPMI of 0 vs. 0.44 in the responder and non-responder groups, respectively (Figure 3).

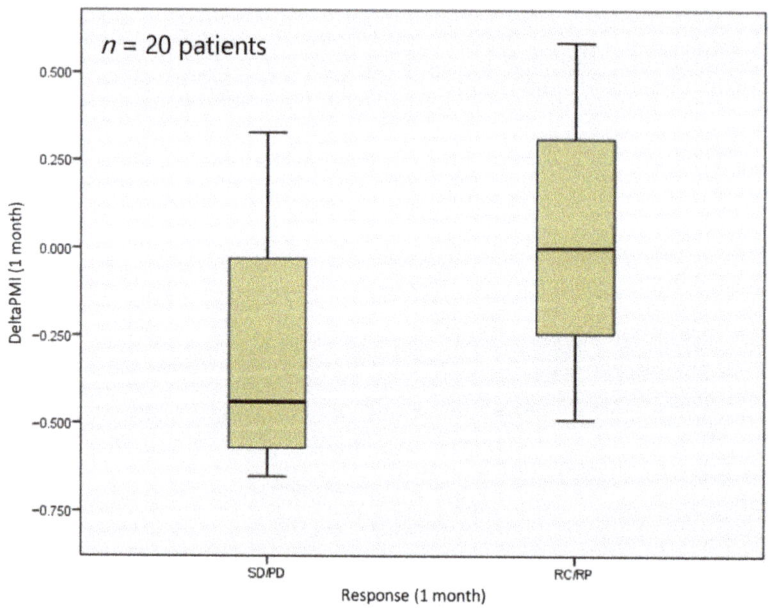


**Figure 3.** DeltaPMI after 1 month evaluated against response to treatment.

At 3 months, however, a statistically significant difference ($p = 0.041$) was observed in terms of sarcopenia status, with a median deltaPMI of 0.12 vs. 0.57 in the responder and non-responder groups, respectively (Figure 4).

A further Mann–Whitney test was conducted to investigate whether deltaPMI could be predictive of a response constant over time. For this purpose, a variable named *bestresp* was introduced and defined as follows: 1 if the response after one month was confirmed after three months and 0 otherwise.

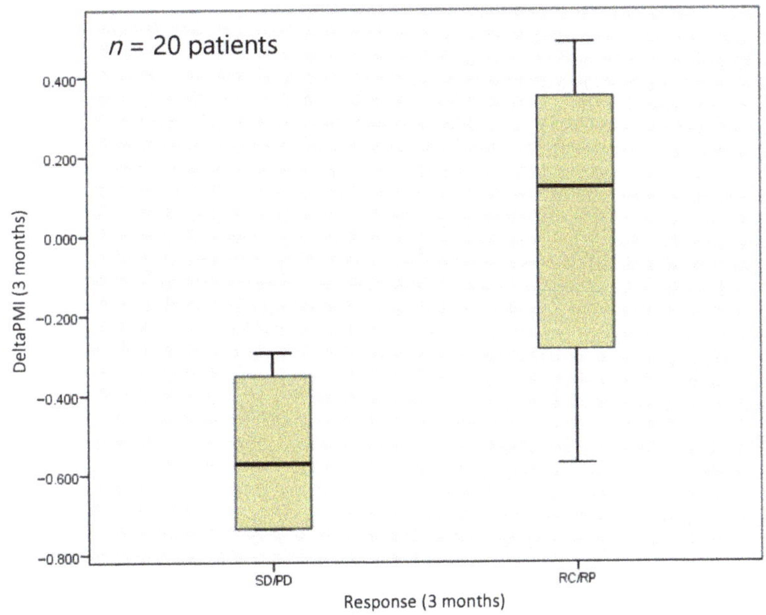


**Figure 4.** DeltaPMI after 3 months evaluated against response to treatment.

No statistically significant relevance ($p = 0.247$) was observed for data collected one month after TARE, probably due to the fact that it is premature to evaluate the radiological response to TARE treatment only one month after the procedure (Figure 5).

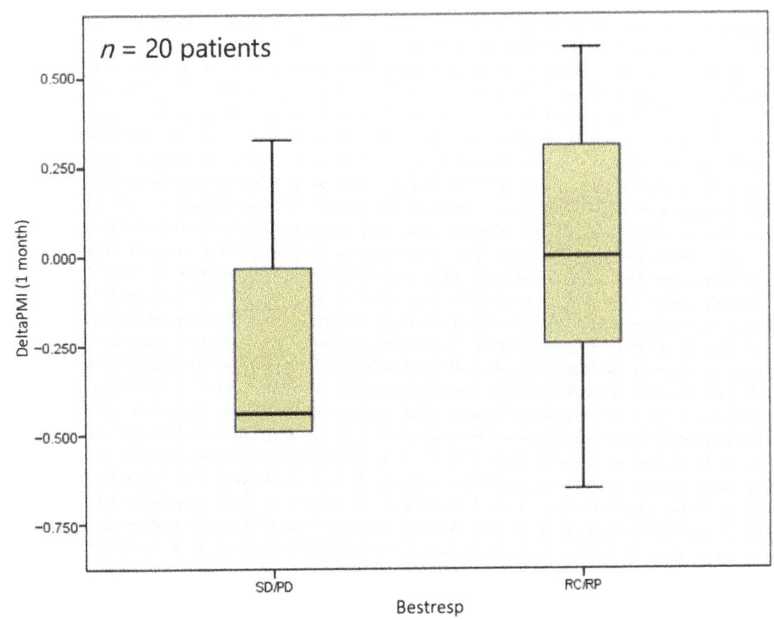


**Figure 5.** DeltaPMI after 1 month evaluated against the bestresp variable.

The same analysis conducted 3 months after TARE showed that deltaPMI can be considered to be a predictive biomarker of local response rate ($p = 0.028$). In particular, we found that a strong negative variation in PMI is associated with a poor response to treatment, with a median deltaPMI of −0.57 in the non-responder and 0.12 in the responder groups, respectively (Figure 6). It was interesting to note that the diagnostic ability for stable or progressive disease of the sarcopenia measurement increased with time after the TARE procedure.

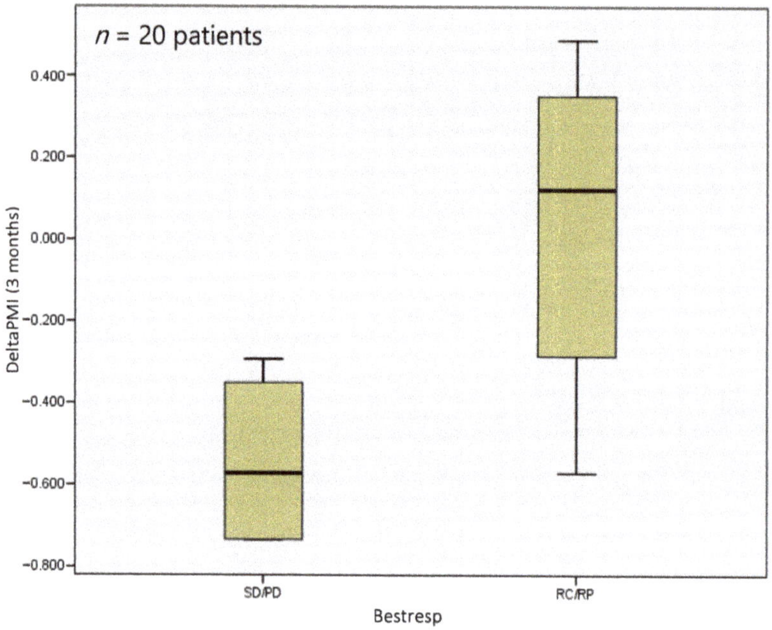


**Figure 6.** DeltaPMI after 3 months evaluated against the bestrep variable.

The ROC analysis was also used to investigate the optimal cut-off of deltaPMI that is statistically relevant in the prediction of a bestresp (i.e., a response to treatment constant over time).

At three months, the deltaPMI value had an AUC = 0.875 ($p = 0.0001$, CIs 0.617 to 0.984). In particular, a PMI variation greater than −0.293 was associated with a bestresp.

This seems to confirm that a small deltaPMI variation is predictive of good treatment. In fact, all 10 patients (100%) who showed a PMI variation greater than the cut-off had a good response to treatment (Fisher's exact test, $p = 0.019$).

## 4. Discussion

Sarcopenia deterioration at three months after TARE treatment with Holmium-166 is a reliable predictor of worse loco-regional response rate in HCC patients.

Sarcopenia has functioned as a predictive element across various clinical scenarios. It has been employed as a predictive factor among patients with HCC [21], including patients undergoing Sorafenib [22,23] or intra-arterial chemoembolization [20], and those pre- or post-transplant [24]. Recently, sarcopenia worsening after TARE treatment with Yttrium-90 has been associated with progressive disease in the early stages [15]. Lastly, with this study, we have determined the association of sarcopenia deterioration at 3 months with TARE-166Ho.

The latest development in radionuclide therapy, Holmium-166, has emerged as a viable substitute for Yttrium-90 in TARE, demonstrating several advantages as previously described. The analysis conducted three months after TARE-166Ho treatment revealed that sarcopenia status could serve as a predictive biomarker for the local response rate ($p = 0.028$). Importantly, our results showed that a decrease in PMI was associated with an unfavorable treatment response, with a median deltaPMI of 0.57 observed in the non-responder group compared to a median value of 0.12 in the responder cohort ($p = 0.041$). Furthermore, we noted an increasing trend in the diagnostic efficacy of sarcopenia measurement for distinguishing stable or progressive disease over the one-to-three-month period following TARE.

This highlights the significance of sarcopenia assessment in effectively predicting the intermediate local outcome following TARE-166Ho, irrespectively of gender differences. Consequently, the deterioration of sarcopenia correlates with a poorer mRECIST score at the intermediate stage.

No statistically significant differences in sarcopenia status were observed at one month post-procedure in either group. This lack of difference is likely due to the premature nature of assessing radiological response to TARE treatment within just one month after the procedure. Additionally, there were no statistically significant distinctions in pre-procedural sarcopenia status between the cohort of patients experiencing progressive disease and those achieving complete response, partial response, or stable disease. This suggests that the initial evaluation of sarcopenia cannot reliably predict unfavorable oncological outcomes following TARE.

Of note, our assessment of TARE treatment response was carried out through CT and MRI or FDG-PET scans, techniques which necessitate a minimum of three–six months to allow for accurate insights into TARE outcomes [25].

In addition to what was previously published regarding the association between sarcopenia worsening and HCC progression at 1 and 3 months after TARE-90Y, this study confirms the same outcomes utilizing Holmium-166 [13]. However, Holmium releases a higher dose rate over a briefer period compared to Y-90, obtaining a faster tumor response and potentially affecting the muscle volume sooner. This allows sarcopenia to be used as a faster predictive index for tumor response.

The divergence in sarcopenia status, identified three months post-procedure through routinely conducted multiphasic CT scans, emerges as a convenient non-invasive predictive biomarker for treatment efficacy, confirming the association between skeletal muscle depletion and a poorer loco-regional response rate. These findings suggest that patients could benefit from early adjustment for skeletal muscle depletion using simple non-invasive methods, which could enhance clinical management by reducing the likelihood of disease progression. Early identification of declining sarcopenia could prompt the implementation of aggressive support protocols. Multimodal approaches, including nutritional support, physical therapy, and medications such as ibuprofen (Menac trial) and selective androgen receptor modulators, as well as ghrelin receptor activation with agonists, are recognized as foundational in managing sarcopenia.

Moreover, the initial sarcopenic status could serve as a guiding factor in selecting a subset of HCC patients undergoing TARE as a preparatory step for liver transplant. This suggests that sarcopenia status could assist in identifying individuals with predictable positive outcomes following transplantation who may benefit from it. Conversely, the early identification of patients at risk of non-responsiveness could be valuable in guiding the timely implementation of systemic therapies. Moreover, the potential of sarcopenia status to predict disease progression could assist in identifying candidates for early TARE re-treatment. Discussions regarding re-treatment often arise in cases where patients tolerated the initial procedure without substantial improvement, though there is no consensus regarding the optimal timing for re-treatment, especially considering the necessary CT/MRI assessment time-frame.

The study has several limitations that need discussion. Foremost, the retrospective nature of the study design precludes the establishment of a randomized framework, which may influence the generalizability of the findings. Secondly, the sample size under analysis was relatively modest; however, given the encouraging results of this pilot study, we hope to continue with a prospective study at our institution, focusing on 166Ho microspheres and sarcopenia, involving a larger sample size. The future trajectory of research would ideally also encompass randomized studies to confirm and further validate these results.

## 5. Conclusions

TARE treatment has firmly established itself as a therapeutic option for patients with locally advanced HCC; more recently, Holmium-166 has introduced new possibilities in this population due to its various advantages. However, assessing the response to TARE treatment in the early stages of follow-up can be challenging. The deterioration of sarcopenia status is a reliable predictor of a worse local response rate at three months after TARE-166Ho, potentially serving as a valuable indicator for identifying patients at early high risk of disease progression. Indeed, the PMI decreased significantly more in the group of poor responders. If our findings are confirmed in larger populations, they could play a pivotal role in the early identification of patients who do not respond to endovascular treatment with Holmium-166 and who may benefit from prompt integrative restorative interventions.

**Author Contributions:** Conceptualization, C.T., N.U., F.C. and G.V.; Methodology, N.U. and M.A.T.; Formal analysis, S.U.; Investigation, L.T.; Resources, G.V.; Data curation, C.T., N.U. and S.U.; Writing—original draft, C.T. and N.U.; Writing—review and editing, F.C. and G.V.; Supervision, L.T. and M.A.T. All authors have read and agreed to the published version of the manuscript.

**Funding:** This research did not receive any specific grant from funding agencies in the public, commercial, or not-for-profit sectors.

**Institutional Review Board Statement:** This is an observational retrospective study and was approved by the Institutional Review Board (Ethical Committee Lazio Area 5) of the "Istituto Regina Elena Istituto di Ricovero e Cura a Carattere Scientifico", with the protocol number code CE RS1561/21(2547).

**Informed Consent Statement:** Informed consent was obtained from all individual participants included in the study.

**Data Availability Statement:** The datasets generated during and/or analyzed during the current study are available from the corresponding author on reasonable request.

**Conflicts of Interest:** The authors declare no conflicts of interest. The funders had no role in the design of the study; in the collection, analyses, or interpretation of data; in the writing of the manuscript; or in the decision to publish the results.

## References

1. Oh, J.H.; Jun, D.W. The latest global burden of liver cancer: A past and present threat. *Clin. Mol. Hepatol.* **2023**, *29*, 355–357. [CrossRef] [PubMed]
2. D'Avola, D.; Lñarrairaegui, M.; Bilbao, J.I.; Martinez-Cuesta, A.; Alegre, F.; Herrero, J.I.; Quiroga, J.; Prieto, J.; Sangro, B. A retrospective comparative analysis of the effect of Y90-radioembolization on the survival of patients with unresectable hepatocellular carcinoma. *Hepatogastroenterology* **2009**, *56*, 1683–1688.
3. Ariel, I.M.; Pack, G.T. Treatment of inoperable cancer of the liver by intra-arterial radioactive isotopes and chemotherapy. *Cancer* **1967**, *20*, 793–804. [CrossRef] [PubMed]
4. Guiu, B.; Garin, E.; Allimant, C.; Edeline, J.; Salem, R. TARE in Hepatocellular Carcinoma: From the Right to the Left of BCLC. *Cardiovasc. Interv. Radiol.* **2022**, *45*, 1599–1607. [CrossRef]
5. Dhondt, E.; Lambert, B.; Hermie, L.; Huyck, L.; Vanlangenhove, P.; Geerts, A.; Verhelst, X.; Aerts, M.; Vanlander, A.; Berrevoet, F.; et al. 90Y Radioembolization versus Drug-eluting Bead Chemoembolization for Unresectable Hepatocellular Carcinoma: Results from the TRACE Phase II Randomized Controlled Trial. *Radiology* **2022**, *303*, 699–710. [CrossRef]
6. Kulik, L.M.; Carr, B.I.; Mulcahy, M.F.; Lewandowski, R.J.; Atassi, B.; Ryu, R.K.; Sato, K.T.; Benson, A.; Nemcek, A.A.; Gates, V.L.; et al. Safety and efficacy of 90Y radiotherapy for hepatocellular carcinoma with and without portal vein thrombosis. *Hepatology* **2008**, *47*, 71–81. [CrossRef]
7. El Fouly, A.; Ertle, J.; El Dorry, A.; Shaker, M.K.; Dechêne, A.; Abdella, H.; Mueller, S.; Barakat, E.; Lauenstein, T.; Bockisch, A.; et al. In intermediate stage hepatocellular carcinoma: Radioembolization with yttrium 90 or chemoembolization? *Liver Int.* **2015**, *35*, 627–635. [CrossRef]

8. Bouvry, C.; Palard, X.; Edeline, J.; Ardisson, V.; Loyer, P.; Garin, E.; Lepareur, N. Transarterial Radioembolization (TARE) Agents beyond 90Y-Microspheres. *BioMed Res. Int.* **2018**, *2018*, 1435302. [CrossRef] [PubMed]
9. Stella, M.; Braat, A.J.A.T.; van Rooij, R.; de Jong, H.W.A.M.; Lam, M.G.E.H. Holmium-166 Radioembolization: Current Status and Future Prospective. *Cardiovasc. Interv. Radiol.* **2022**, *45*, 1634–1645. [CrossRef]
10. van de Maat, G.H.; Seevinck, P.R.; Elschot, M.; Smits, M.L.J.; de Leeuw, H.; van Het Schip, A.D.; Vente, M.A.D.; Zonnenberg, B.A.; de Jong, H.W.A.M.; Lam, M.G.E.H.; et al. MRI-based biodistribution assessment of holmium-166 poly(L-lactic acid) microspheres after radioembolisation. *Eur. Radiol.* **2013**, *23*, 827–835. [CrossRef]
11. Reinders, M.T.M.; van Erpecum, K.J.; Smits, M.L.J.; Braat, A.J.A.T.; de Bruijne, J.; Bruijnen, R.; Sprengers, D.; de Man, R.A.; Vegt, E.; IJzermans, J.N.M.; et al. Safety and Efficacy of 166Ho Radioembolization in Hepatocellular Carcinoma: The HEPAR Primary Study. *J. Nucl. Med.* **2022**, *63*, 1891–1898. [CrossRef] [PubMed]
12. Drescher, R.; Köhler, A.; Seifert, P.; Aschenbach, R.; Ernst, T.; Rauchfuß, F.; Freesmeyer, M. Clinical Results of Transarterial Radioembolization (TARE) with Holmium-166 Microspheres in the Multidisciplinary Oncologic Treatment of Patients with Primary and Secondary Liver Cancer. *Biomedicines* **2023**, *11*, 1831. [CrossRef] [PubMed]
13. Perisetti, A.; Goyal, H.; Yendala, R.; Chandan, S.; Tharian, B.; Thandassery, R.B. Sarcopenia in hepatocellular carcinoma: Current knowledge and future directions. *World J. Gastroenterol.* **2022**, *28*, 432–448. [CrossRef] [PubMed]
14. Palazzoadriano, M.; Albano, V.; Bellanca, L.; Latteri, S.; Valdes, L.; Mangiameli, S. Modifications induced in the renin-angiotensin-aldo-sterone system of rats by alpha-blocking drugs. *Pharmacol. Res. Commun.* **1978**, *10*, 925–937. [CrossRef] [PubMed]
15. Vallati, G.E.; Trobiani, C.; Teodoli, L.; Lai, Q.; Cappelli, F.; Ungania, S.; Catalano, C.; Lucatelli, P. Sarcopenia Worsening One Month after Transarterial Radioembolization Predicts Progressive Disease in Patients with Advanced Hepatocellular Carcinoma. *Biology* **2021**, *10*, 728. [CrossRef] [PubMed]
16. Badran, H.; Elsabaawy, M.M.; Ragab, A.; Aly, R.A.; Alsebaey, A.; Sabry, A. Baseline Sarcopenia is Associated with Lack of Response to Therapy, Liver Decompensation and High Mortality in Hepatocellular Carcinoma Patients. *Asian Pac. J. Cancer Prev.* **2020**, *21*, 3285–3290. [CrossRef] [PubMed]
17. Xu, L.; Jing, Y.; Zhao, C.; Zhang, Q.; Zhao, X.; Yang, J.; Wu, L.; Yang, Y. Preoperative computed tomography-assessed skeletal muscle index is a novel prognostic factor in patients with hepatocellular carcinoma following hepatectomy: A meta-analysis. *J. Gastrointest. Oncol.* **2020**, *11*, 1040–1053. [CrossRef] [PubMed]
18. Cheng, T.-Y.; Lee, P.-C.; Chen, Y.-T.; Chao, Y.; Hou, M.-C.; Huang, Y.-H. Pre-sarcopenia determines post-progression outcomes in advanced hepatocellular carcinoma after sorafenib failure. *Sci. Rep.* **2020**, *10*, 18375. [CrossRef]
19. Santilli, V.; Bernetti, A.; Mangone, M.; Paoloni, M. Clinical definition of sarcopenia. *Clin. Cases Miner. Bone Metab.* **2014**, *11*, 177–180. [CrossRef]
20. Fujita, M.; Takahashi, A.; Hayashi, M.; Okai, K.; Abe, K.; Ohira, H. Skeletal muscle volume loss during transarterial chemoembolization predicts poor prognosis in patients with hepatocellular carcinoma. *Hepatol. Res.* **2019**, *49*, 778–786. [CrossRef]
21. Chang, K.-V.; Chen, J.-D.; Wu, W.-T.; Huang, K.-C.; Hsu, C.-T.; Han, D.-S. Association between Loss of Skeletal Muscle Mass and Mortality and Tumor Recurrence in Hepatocellular Carcinoma: A Systematic Review and Meta-Analysis. *Liver Cancer* **2018**, *7*, 90–103. [CrossRef] [PubMed]
22. Takada, H.; Kurosaki, M.; Nakanishi, H.; Takahashi, Y.; Itakura, J.; Tsuchiya, K.; Yasui, Y.; Tamaki, N.; Takaura, K.; Komiyama, Y.; et al. Impact of pre-sarcopenia in sorafenib treatment for advanced hepatocellular carcinoma. *PLoS ONE* **2018**, *13*, e0198812. [CrossRef] [PubMed]
23. Yamashima, M.; Miyaaki, H.; Honda, T.; Shibata, H.; Miuma, S.; Taura, N.; Nakao, K. Significance of psoas muscle thickness as an indicator of muscle atrophy in patients with hepatocellular carcinoma treated with sorafenib. *Mol. Clin. Oncol.* **2017**, *7*, 449–453. [CrossRef] [PubMed]
24. Ahmadzadehfar, H.; Duan, H.; Haug, A.R.; Walrand, S.; Hoffmann, M. The role of SPECT/CT in radioembolization of liver tumours. *Eur. J. Nucl. Med. Mol. Imaging* **2014**, *41* (Suppl. S1), S115–S124. [CrossRef]
25. Adcock, C.S.; Florez, E.; Zand, K.A.; Patel, A.; Howard, C.M.; Fatemi, A. Assessment of Treatment Response Following Yttrium-90 Transarterial Radioembolization of Liver Malignancies. *Cureus* **2018**, *10*, e2895. [CrossRef]

Journal of *Personalized Medicine*

MDPI

*Communication*

# Lateral Pectoral Nerve Identification through Ultrasound-Guided Methylene Blue Injection during Selective Peripheral Neurectomy for Shoulder Spasticity: Proposal for a New Procedure

**Paolo Zerbinati [1], Jonathan Bemporad [1], Andrea Massimiani [2], Edoardo Bianchini [2], Davide Mazzoli [3], Davide Glorioso [1], Giuseppe della Vecchia [4], Antonio De Luca [5] and Paolo De Blasiis [5,*]**

[1] Neuro-Orthopedic Unit, Sol et Salus Hospital, 47922 Rimini, Italy; j.bemporad@soletsalus.com (J.B.); d.glorioso@soletsalus.com (D.G.)

[2] Department of Neuroscience, Mental Health and Sensory Organs (NESMOS), Sapienza University of Rome, 00189 Rome, Italy; andrea.massimiani@uniroma.it (A.M.); edoardo.bianchini@uniroma1.it (E.B.)

[3] Gait and Motion Analysis Laboratory, Sol et Salus Hospital, 47992 Rimini, Italy; d.mazzoli@soletsalus.com

[4] Department of Women, Child, General and Specialistic Surgery, University of Campania "L. Vanvitelli", 80138 Naples, Italy; dellavecchia-g@libero.it

[5] Section of Human Anatomy, Department of Mental and Physical Health and Preventive Medicine, University of Campania "Luigi Vanvitelli", Via Luciano Armanni, 5, 80138 Naples, Italy; antonio.deluca@unicampania.it

* Correspondence: paolo.deblasiis@unicampania.it; Tel.: +39-081-458225

**Abstract:** Internally rotated and adducted shoulder is a common posture in upper limb spasticity. Selective peripheral neurectomy is a useful and viable surgical technique to ameliorate spasticity, and the lateral pectoral nerve (LPN) could be a potential good target to manage shoulder spasticity presenting with internal rotation. However, there are some limitations related to this procedure, such as potential anatomical variability and the necessity of intraoperative surgical exploration to identify the target nerve requiring wide surgical incisions. This could result in higher post-surgical discomfort for the patient. Therefore, the aim of our study was to describe a modification of the traditional selective peripheral neurectomy procedure of the LPN through the perioperative ultrasound-guided marking of the target nerve with methylene blue. The details of the localization and marking procedure are described, as well as the surgical technique of peripheral selective neurectomy and the potential advantages in terms of nerve localization, surgical precision and patients' post-surgical discomfort. We suggest that the proposed modified procedure could be a valid technique to address some current limitations and move the surgical treatment of spasticity toward increasingly tailored management due to the ease of nerve identification, the possibility of handling potential anatomical variability and the resulting smaller surgical incisions.

**Keywords:** spasticity; shoulder spasticity; selective neurectomy; functional surgery; lateral pectoral nerve; ultrasonography; methylene blue

## 1. Introduction

Spasticity is a common and complex motor phenomenon following upper motor neuron injury [1] characterized by muscle hyperactivity, with velocity-dependent hypertonia and abnormally increased tendon jerks [2]. Among involved body segments, upper limb spasticity (ULS) is common in post-stroke patients [3], with over 40% of patients reporting it [4,5], and leads to a potentially high functional limitation for patients [6,7]. Several pattern and postures have been described for ULS [8] and the involvement of the shoulder, in particular with internally rotated and adducted arm posture, is present in the vast majority of patients presenting with ULS [8]. Moreover, from 8% to 13% patients with post-stroke spasticity suffer from shoulder pain, a percentage that increases to over 25% in presence of disabling spasticity [9].

The severity of spasticity can vary greatly and, over time, this condition can lead to retractions, contractures, deformities, pressure ulcers and skin maceration [2], with a high impact on patients' quality of life [10,11]. Therefore, the prompt identification and effective management of spasticity is crucial to assuring the best possible outcome for patients. To this end, several treatment options are available, including pharmacological therapy, rehabilitative treatment, chemodenervation techniques (e.g., botulinum toxin injection, nerve blocks) and surgery [12]. Among this latter option, possible strategies for spasticity management include selective and hyperselective peripheral neurectomies [13].

Peripheral neurectomies consist of the partial excision of the fibers of a motor nerve innervating spastic muscles [14]. The first one was described by Stoffel and colleagues [15] and then by Brunelli and Brunelli [16], becoming increasingly common procedures. While their origins date back to the first decades of the 20th century, selective peripheral neurectomy has received growing attention in recent years since this procedure has been demonstrated to mitigate muscle spasticity, particularly in lower limbs [17–21]. Based on this evidence, in fact, an international, interdisciplinary Delphi panel recently included selective neurectomies among the treatments for poststroke equinovarus foot deformities [22].

Although no recommendations exist for upper limbs, several studies demonstrated the effectiveness of selective peripheral neurectomy in ULS as well [13,14,18,23–27]. Regarding shoulder spasticity, only very few papers exist. In one study from Lin and colleagues [23], hyperselective neurectomy of thoracodorsal nerve was demonstrated to be effective in the treatment of shoulder spasticity. In another retrospective study, Sitthinamsuwan and collaborators [27] demonstrated the efficacy of selective neurotomy in the treatment of refractory ULS, including 14 patients undergoing pectoral nerve neurotomy. Lateral pectoral nerve (LPN) is a good potential target when surgically treating shoulder spasticity presenting with internal rotation. This nerve, indeed, innervates the pectoralis major muscle [28], one of the primary targets in shoulder spasticity management using botulinum toxin [29]. Moreover, diagnostic LPN nerve block has recently been proposed as part of an algorithm to evaluate hemiplegic shoulder pain [30].

During selective peripheral neurectomy of the LPN, after surgical incision in the infraclavicular fossa and partial reflection of clavipectoral fascia and pectoralis major, surgical exploration is carried out, and the nerve is located using electrical stimulation while observing the contraction of the pectoralis major. After locating the nerve motor fibers, a partial section is performed [27].

However, there are some limitations related to this procedure: (i) potential anatomical variability [31–33], which could increase surgical operative time and difficulty in locating the nerve; (ii) the fact that in order to perform surgical exploration, a sufficiently wide surgical incision is necessary; and (iii) the necessity of intraoperative search and identification of the nerve. This could also result in higher post-surgical discomfort for the patient.

## 2. Materials and Methods

The aim of this paper is to describe a modification of the traditional selective peripheral neurectomy procedure of the LPN through the perioperative ultrasound-guided marking of the target nerve with methylene blue. The details of the localization and marking procedure are described, as well as the surgical technique of peripheral selective neurectomy and the potential advantages in terms of nerve localization, surgical precision and patients' post-surgical discomfort.

## 3. Results

### 3.1. Patient Selection and Indications

Patients with shoulder spasticity presenting with internally rotated and adducted arm posture could have an indication to undergo the selective peripheral neurectomy of the LPN described in this paper. The proposed technique is primarily described for adult patients with acquired spasticity; however, this could, in principle, be extended to pediatric patients as well since no contraindication to the use of methylene blue is present in this population and selective neurectomies are performed in children to treat ULS [24]. An assessment of patient motivation and cognition could be performed during each patient's evaluation. However, since several conditions leading to spasticity could also involve cognitive impairment, cognitive deficit should not be considered an absolute contraindication to the procedure as long as the patient can cope with a surgical procedure and the postoperative regimen. A goal attainment scale could be included in each patient's evaluation in order to guarantee a patient-centric approach. Since selective peripheral neurectomy is only effective on spasticity and has no effect on muscle or joint contractures, if the presence of a structural alteration such as those previously mentioned is suspected, a diagnostic nerve block of the LPN might be performed in order to predict the outcome of the surgical procedure. This is similar to the recommendation for the management of poststroke equinovarus foot deformities proposed by Salga and colleagues [22]. In the case of limited or no response to the diagnostic nerve block, other management strategies, such as functional surgery (e.g., tendon elongment, tenothomies, etc.) could be taken into consideration. Known hypersensitivity to methylene blue is a contraindication to this procedure and should lead to the choice of an alternative technique. General contraindications for surgery in patients with ULS linked to the procedure or anesthesia also apply to this technique, such as dystonia or other movement disorders, a lack of patient compliance, unrealistic expectations or high intraoperative risk, as judged by an anesthesiologist and surgeon.

### 3.2. US-Guided Nerve Localization and Marking

A sonographic unit coupled with a linear multifrequency probe is used for ultrasonographic guidance. With the patient in a supine position, the operator positions themselves on the same side as the target muscle. The LPN is located at the brachial plexus origin in the subclavian region, laterally to the hemiclavear line and approximately 3 cm below the clavicle, by positioning the probe parallel to the direction of the pectoralis major fibers. The nerve is then followed in the cranio-caudal direction, between the pectoralis major and pectoralis minor muscles, until the motor fibers for the pectoralis major muscle are identified (Figure 1).

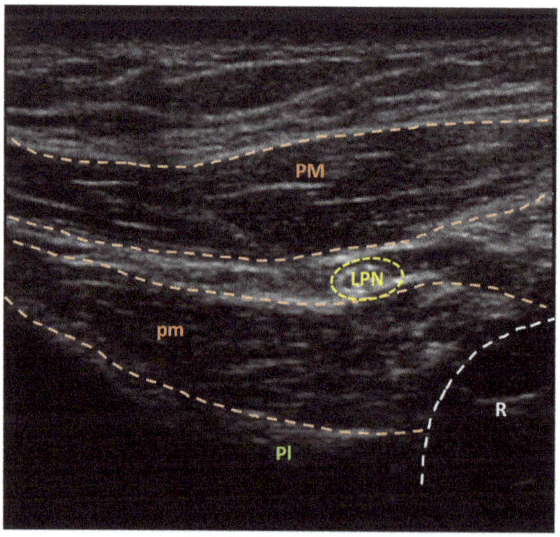


**Figure 1.** Ultrasonographic visualization of lateral pectoral nerve (yellow circle) before methylene blue injection. LPN: lateral pectoral nerve; Pl: pleura; PM: pectoralis major muscle; pm: pectoralis minor muscle; R: rib. A sonographic unit (Sonoscape X3, Sonoscape Europe s.r.l., Rome, Italy), coupled with a linear multifrequency probe (5–14 MHz, L741, Sonoscape Europe s.r.l., Rome, Italy), was used for ultrasonographic guidance.

The exact point at which the motor fibers detach from the main nerve trunk can be easily identified by performing slow cranio-caudal and caudo-cranial probe movements following the nerve course. This is crucial since the branching point is the site at which the neurectomy will be carried out.

After identifying the motor fiber origin location, a needle electrode connected to an electro-stimulator is inserted, in aseptic conditions, under ultrasound guidance and positioned in the proximity of the nerve previously identified. A current of 0.8–1 mA at the nerve site is then used to confirm the identified nerve by eliciting a contraction in the pectoralis major muscle. Once an adequate muscle contraction is evoked, the intensity of the stimulus is progressively reduced until the minimum possible stimulus capable of determining visible muscle contraction is reached (usually around 0.2–0.4 mA).

Thus, 0.8–1.2 mL of methylene blue solution 1% (Figure 2) is injected around the target nerve (Figure 3).

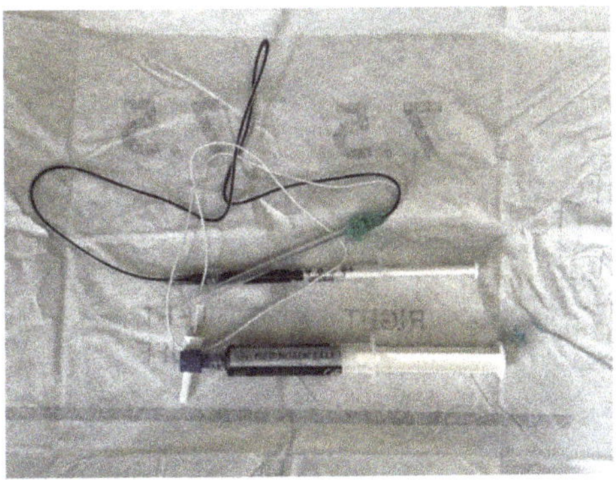

**Figure 2.** Syringe containing methylene blue solution 1% connected to a needle electrode.

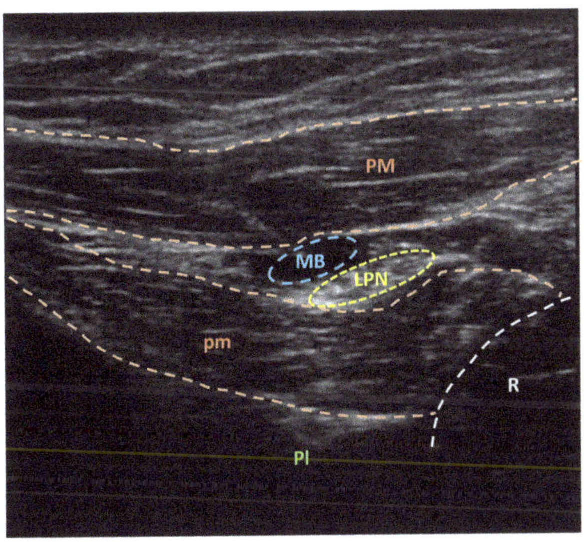


**Figure 3.** Ultrasonographic visualization of lateral pectoral nerve (yellow circle) after methylene blue injection (blue circle). LPN: lateral pectoral nerve; MB: methylene blue; Pl: pleura; PM: pectoralis major muscle; pm: pectoralis minor muscle; R: rib. A sonographic unit (Sonoscape X3, Sonoscape Europe s.r.l., Rome, Italy), coupled with a linear multifrequency probe (5–14 MHz, L741, Sonoscape Europe s.r.l., Rome, Italy), was used for ultrasonographic guidance.

### 3.3. Setup

Selective neurectomy is performed with the patient in a supine position under general anesthesia. Paralysis is contraindicated because of the need for muscle contraction following intraoperative nerve stimulation.

### 3.4. Exposure

After general anesthesia, a transverse lateral subclavicular incision of approximately 2 cm is made at the site at which the branching point was identified, using the needle entrance point as a guide. It is usually 2–3 cm below the lateral third of the clavicula but can vary from individual to individual. Hemostasis is performed, and partial reflection of the great pectoralis is carried out, exposing the pectoralis minor and the LPN lying in the plane between the two muscles. The nerve branch can be easily identified at this level by the methylene blue marking. A silicone elastic loop is then placed around the nerve to isolate it (Figure 4).

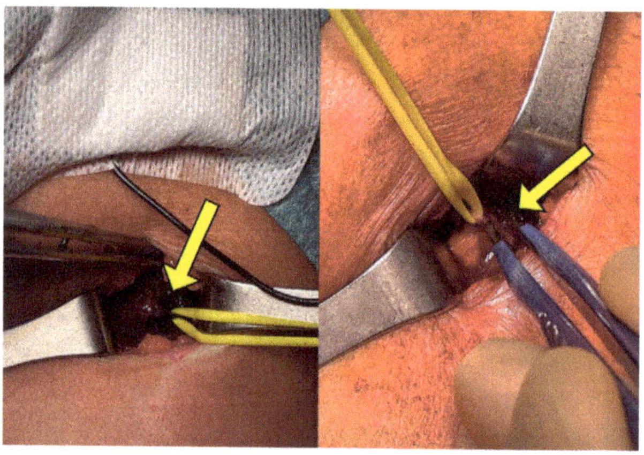

**Figure 4.** LPN visualization during surgical procedure with silicone loop placed for nerve isolation. The target nerve is located through the methylene blue marking colorization (arrow).

An intraoperative electrostimulation is then used to confirm the identified nerve (Figure 5) by observing the contraction of the pectoralis major muscle.

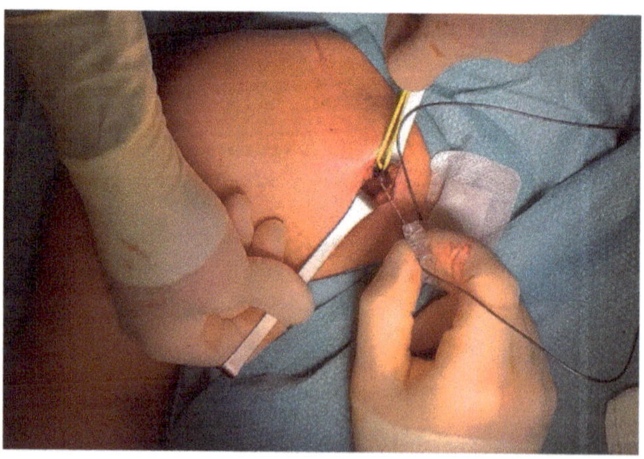

**Figure 5.** Electrostimulation during surgical procedure to confirm the identified nerve using methylene blue marking.

### 3.5. Selective Peripheral Neurectomy

Once the isolated nerve is confirmed to comprise the target motor fibers of the LPN, the selective peripheral neurectomy is carried out by performing a microsurgical partial section of the motor nerve fibers. The epineurium is incised along the long axis of the nerve, and 50 to 75% of all fascicles are resected from the main trunk, depending on the extent of spasticity and the desired outcome (Figure 6).

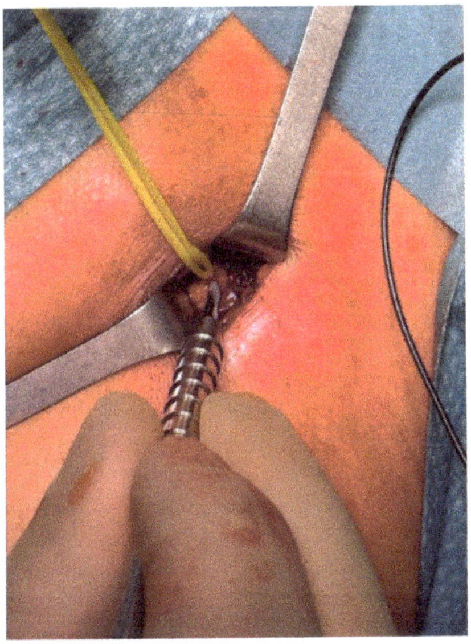

**Figure 6.** Fiber partial section of the LPN marked with methylene blue during selective neurectomy procedure.

Coagulation of the proximal and distal stumps is performed in order to prevent nerve regrowth and to slow sprouting.

### 3.6. Closure and Postoperative Care

Once the neurectomy is completed, the surgical wound is sutured and the procedure is concluded. Postoperative care consists of a soft, nonadherent dressing until the wound is healed. Gentle passive stretching and active exercises of the involved muscles are subsequently initiated according to patient conditions.

## 4. Discussion

The aim of this paper is to describe a modification to the traditional selective peripheral neurectomy procedure of the LPN through the perioperative ultrasound-guided marking of the target nerve with methylene blue.

The use of elective peripheral neurectomy to mitigate muscle spasticity has received growing attention in recent years. While most evidence supported its use in lower limbs [17–21] and a recently developed recommendation included selective neurectomies among treatments for post-stroke equinovarus foot deformities [22], no recommendations exist for upper limbs. However the effectiveness of selective peripheral neurectomies to treat ULS has been reported [13,14,18,23–27]. In our proposed technique, 50–75% of nerve fascicles are excised during the selective peripheral neurectomy. There is no total agreement on what percentage of the nerve needs to be resected, and this has critical implications for the recurrences that can occur several months after surgery. Sprouting from adjacent axonal endings has been linked to reinnervation and, for this reason, several authors recommended the excision of a relevant percentage of fascicles. Brunelli and Brunelli preformed the excision of around two-thirds of fascicles [16], Maarrawi et al. described the resection of 50% to 80% of the isolated motor branches paired with proximal coagulation to prevent regrowth [34]; Puligopu and Purhoit described the resection of one-third to three-quarters of the motor branches for individual muscles [35]. Similarly, Fouad reported the resection of 50% to 80% of the isolated motor branches of fascicles [36], and, finally, Leclercq described the excision of approximately two-thirds of each nerve branch at the level of the motor branches [24].

It emerges that a detailed knowledge of anatomy is essential in order to plan the operative act; therefore, the literature stresses the concept that guidance techniques and methods to improve nerve branch identification during dissection are crucial [37].

Our work falls into this line of research by using methylene blue to mark target nerve branches during selective peripheral neurectomy. The use of methylene blue as a surgical marker is not new. In fact, previous studies reported its use as a surgical marker to identify parathyroid glands [38] and during lung [39] and abdominal surgery [40]. Moreover, in our experience, the use of methylene blue did not constitute an obstacle to the surgeon's view due to tissue soiling, and reported local adverse events linked to methylene blue toxicity are extremely rare and usually follow more demolitive surgeries such as breast and colon surgeries using higher doses and different dilutions [41].

Several advantages could arise from the proposed nerve marking. The first advantage of the US-guided perioperative identification and marking of the LPN is handling potential anatomical variability. Indeed, the LPN arises most frequently with two branches from the anterior divisions of the upper and middle plexus trunks. However, although anatomical variability seems to be less than in other districts, some variations are described, such as emergence as a single root from the lateral cord or emergence only from middle or upper trunks [37–39]. Anatomical variability could result in difficulties in reliably locating the nerve, increases in surgical operating time and potentially greater post-surgical discomfort for patients. To this end, this procedure has the potential to overcome this limitation since the LPN is easily identified through methylene blue colorization.

Secondly, the ease of nerve identification and the possibility of using the needle entrance hole as an anatomical landmark could also limit the need for surgical exploration, thus reducing the necessity of wider incisions and longer surgical operative time. Figure 7 shows a comparison of surgical incisions in both traditional and modified LPN selective peripheral neurectomy procedures. A smaller surgical wound will likely result in reduced patient discomfort, faster recovery and the reduced occurrence of postoperative complications.

Finally, it is important to underline that the addition of methylene blue marking will hardly affect the selective peripheral neurectomy procedure's time and complexity. Indeed, as discussed above, the procedure will likely lead to a reduction in operative time and greater surgical efficiency. Moreover, nerve identification thorough electrical stimulation is routinely performed in the classical procedure, and the marking phase only adds the injection step, which does not require specific expertise or equipment other than a needle electrode suitable for injection and the methylene blue solution.

Given all these considerations, the proposed modified LPN selective peripheral neurectomy with the use of a perioperative US-guided methylene blue injection could be a valid technique to address some current limitations and move the surgical treatment of spasticity toward increasingly tailored and personalized management. Moreover, this technique can be applied to other districts in which anatomical variability could be a more difficult aspect to address. Future studies are warranted to evaluate the efficacy and the safety profile of this procedure and compare it to the traditional technique.

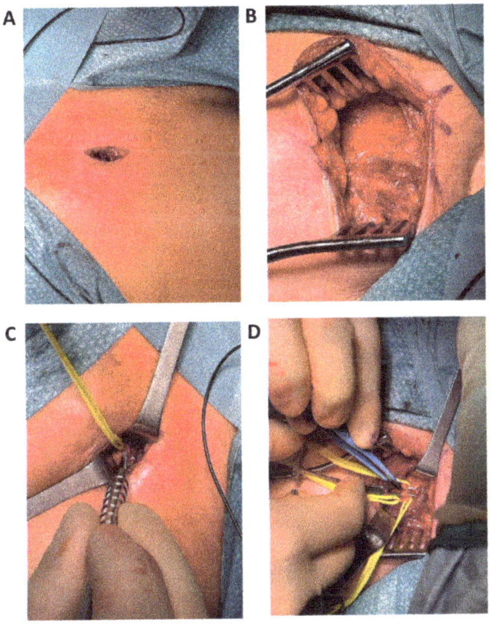


**Figure 7.** Comparison of surgical incision and intraoperative surgical wound in the proposed procedure with methylene blue injection (**A**,**C**) and in a traditional LPN neurectomy (**B**,**D**).

**Author Contributions:** Conceptualization, methodology and validation, P.Z. and J.B.; formal analysis, investigation, resource and data curation, all authors; visualization and writing—original draft preparation, E.B., J.B., P.Z., P.D.B., A.M., G.d.V., D.M. and D.G.; writing—review and editing, all authors; supervision and project administration, P.D.B., A.M. and A.D.L. All authors have read and agreed to the published version of the manuscript.

**Funding:** This research received no external funding.

**Institutional Review Board Statement:** Not applicable.

**Informed Consent Statement:** Not applicable.

**Data Availability Statement:** Not applicable. A novel procedure is described and there is no data.

**Conflicts of Interest:** The authors declare no conflicts of interest.

## References

1. Sheean, G. The Pathophysiology of Spasticity. *Eur. J. Neurol.* **2002**, *9* (Suppl. S1), 3–9; dicussion 53–61. [CrossRef] [PubMed]
2. Kheder, A.; Nair, K.P.S. Spasticity: Pathophysiology, Evaluation and Management. *Pract. Neurol.* **2012**, *12*, 289–298. [CrossRef] [PubMed]
3. Sommerfeld, D.K.; Gripenstedt, U.; Welmer, A.-K. Spasticity after Stroke: An Overview of Prevalence, Test Instruments, and Treatments. *Am. J. Phys. Med. Rehabil.* **2012**, *91*, 814–820. [CrossRef] [PubMed]
4. Lundström, E.; Terént, A.; Borg, J. Prevalence of Disabling Spasticity 1 Year after First-Ever Stroke. *Eur. J. Neurol.* **2008**, *15*, 533–539. [CrossRef] [PubMed]
5. Wissel, J.; Manack, A.; Brainin, M. Toward an Epidemiology of Poststroke Spasticity. *Neurology* **2013**, *80*, S13–S19. [CrossRef] [PubMed]
6. Urban, P.P.; Wolf, T.; Uebele, M.; Marx, J.J.; Vogt, T.; Stoeter, P.; Bauermann, T.; Weibrich, C.; Vucurevic, G.D.; Schneider, A.; et al. Occurence and Clinical Predictors of Spasticity after Ischemic Stroke. *Stroke* **2010**, *41*, 2016–2020. [CrossRef]
7. Katoozian, L.; Tahan, N.; Zoghi, M.; Bakhshayesh, B. The Onset and Frequency of Spasticity After First Ever Stroke. *J. Natl. Med. Assoc.* **2018**, *110*, 547–552. [CrossRef] [PubMed]
8. Hefter, H.; Jost, W.H.; Reissig, A.; Zakine, B.; Bakheit, A.M.; Wissel, J. Classification of Posture in Poststroke Upper Limb Spasticity: A Potential Decision Tool for Botulinum Toxin A Treatment? *Int. J. Rehabil. Res.* **2012**, *35*, 227–233. [CrossRef]

9. Menoux, D.; Jousse, M.; Quintaine, V.; Tlili, L.; Yelnik, A.P. Decrease in Post-Stroke Spasticity and Shoulder Pain Prevalence over the Last 15 Years. *Ann. Phys. Rehabil. Med.* **2019**, *62*, 403–408. [CrossRef]
10. Fheodoroff, K.; Rekand, T.; Medeiros, L.; Koßmehl, P.; Wissel, J.; Bensmail, D.; Scheschonka, A.; Flatau-Baqué, B.; Simon, O.; Dressler, D.; et al. Quality of Life in Subjects with Upper- and Lower-Limb Spasticity Treated with incobotulinumtoxinA. *Health Qual. Life Outcomes* **2020**, *18*, 51. [CrossRef]
11. Doan, Q.V.; Brashear, A.; Gillard, P.J.; Varon, S.F.; Vandenburgh, A.M.; Turkel, C.C.; Elovic, E.P. Relationship between Disability and Health-Related Quality of Life and Caregiver Burden in Patients with Upper Limb Poststroke Spasticity. *PM&R.* **2012**, *4*, 4–10. [CrossRef]
12. Chang, E.; Ghosh, N.; Yanni, D.; Lee, S.; Alexandru, D.; Mozaffar, T. A Review of Spasticity Treatments: Pharmacological and Interventional Approaches. *Crit. Rev. Phys. Rehabil. Med.* **2013**, *25*, 11–22. [CrossRef] [PubMed]
13. Hashemi, M.; Sturbois-Nachef, N.; Keenan, M.A.; Winston, P. Surgical Approaches to Upper Limb Spasticity in Adult Patients: A Literature Review. *Front. Rehabil. Sci.* **2021**, *2*, 709969. [CrossRef] [PubMed]
14. Gras, M.; Leclercq, C. Spasticity and Hyperselective Neurectomy in the Upper Limb. *Hand Surg. Rehabil.* **2017**, *36*, 391–401. [CrossRef]
15. Stoffel, A. The treatment of spastic contractures. *JBJS* **1913**, *s2–s10*, 611.
16. Brunelli, G.; Brunelli, F. Partial Selective Denervation in Spastic Palsies (Hyponeurotization). *Microsurgery* **1983**, *4*, 221–224. [CrossRef]
17. Sindou, M.; Mertens, P. Selective Neurotomy of the Tibial Nerve for Treatment of the Spastic Foot. *Neurosurgery* **1988**, *23*, 738–744. [CrossRef]
18. Mahan, M.A.; Eli, I.; Hamrick, F.; Abou-Al-Shaar, H.; Shingleton, R.; Tucker Balun, K.; Edgley, S.R. Highly Selective Partial Neurectomies for Spasticity: A Single-Center Experience. *Neurosurgery* **2021**, *89*, 827–835. [CrossRef]
19. Emamhadi, M.; Alijani, B.; Haghani Dogahe, M.; Emamhadi, A. Hyper-Selective Neurectomy for Knee Flexion Spasticity: Anatomic Bases and Surgical Technique. *Surg. Radiol. Anat.* **2023**, *45*, 201–205. [CrossRef]
20. Bollens, B.; Gustin, T.; Stoquart, G.; Detrembleur, C.; Lejeune, T.; Deltombe, T. A Randomized Controlled Trial of Selective Neurotomy versus Botulinum Toxin for Spastic Equinovarus Foot after Stroke. *Neurorehabil Neural Repair.* **2013**, *27*, 695–703. [CrossRef]
21. Bollens, B.; Deltombe, T.; Detrembleur, C.; Gustin, T.; Stoquart, G.; Lejeune, T.M. Effects of Selective Tibial Nerve Neurotomy as a Treatment for Adults Presenting with Spastic Equinovarus Foot: A Systematic Review. *J. Rehabil. Med.* **2011**, *43*, 277–282. [CrossRef]
22. Salga, M.; Gatin, L.; Deltombe, T.; Gustin, T.; Carda, S.; Marque, P.; Winston, P.; Reebye, R.; Wein, T.; Esquenazi, A.; et al. International Recommendations to Manage Poststroke Equinovarus Foot Deformity Validated by a Panel of Experts Using Delphi. *Arch. Phys. Med. Rehabil.* **2022**, *104*, 372–379. [CrossRef]
23. Lin, W.; Li, T.; Qi, W.; Shen, Y.; Xu, W. Hyperselective Neurectomy of Thoracodorsal Nerve for Treatment of the Shoulder Spasticity: Anatomical Study and Preliminary Clinical Results. *Acta Neurochir.* **2023**, *165*, 1179–1188. [CrossRef] [PubMed]
24. Leclercq, C.; Perruisseau-Carrier, A.; Gras, M.; Panciera, P.; Fulchignoni, C.; Fulchignoni, M. Hyperselective Neurectomy for the Treatment of Upper Limb Spasticity in Adults and Children: A Prospective Study. *J. Hand Surg.* **2021**, *46*, 708–716. [CrossRef]
25. Yong, L.Y.; Wong, C.H.L.; Gaston, M.; Lam, W.L. The Role of Selective Peripheral Neurectomy in the Treatment of Upper Limb Spasticity. *J. Hand Surg.* **2018**, *23*, 181–191. [CrossRef] [PubMed]
26. Heredia-Gutierrez, A.; Carbarin-Carbarin, M.E.; Torres-Garcia, S.; Gonzalez-Carranza, V.; de Leon, F.C.-P. The Utility of Selective Partial Neurectomy of the Musculocutaneous Nerve in Children with Bilateral Spastic Elbow. *Childs Nerv. Syst.* **2023**, *39*, 3509–3514. [CrossRef] [PubMed]
27. Sitthinamsuwan, B.; Chanvanitkulchai, K.; Phonwijit, L.; Nunta-Aree, S.; Kumthornthip, W.; Ploypetch, T. Surgical Outcomes of Microsurgical Selective Peripheral Neurotomy for Intractable Limb Spasticity. *Stereotact. Funct. Neurosurg.* **2013**, *91*, 248–257. [CrossRef] [PubMed]
28. Rea, P. Chapter 2—Upper Limb Nerve Supply. In *Essential Clinically Applied Anatomy of the Peripheral Nervous System in the Limbs*; Rea, P., Ed.; Academic Press: Cambridge, MA, USA, 2015; pp. 41–100. ISBN 978-0-12-803062-2.
29. Simpson, D.M.; Hallett, M.; Ashman, E.J.; Comella, C.L.; Green, M.W.; Gronseth, G.S.; Armstrong, M.J.; Gloss, D.; Potrebic, S.; Jankovic, J.; et al. Practice Guideline Update Summary: Botulinum Neurotoxin for the Treatment of Blepharospasm, Cervical Dystonia, Adult Spasticity, and Headache: Report of the Guideline Development Subcommittee of the American Academy of Neurology. *Neurology* **2016**, *86*, 1818–1826. [CrossRef]
30. Fitterer, J.W.; Picelli, A.; Winston, P. A Novel Approach to New-Onset Hemiplegic Shoulder Pain With Decreased Range of Motion Using Targeted Diagnostic Nerve Blocks: The ViVe Algorithm. *Front. Neurol.* **2021**, *12*, 668370. [CrossRef]
31. Porzionato, A.; Macchi, V.; Stecco, C.; Loukas, M.; Tubbs, R.S.; De Caro, R. Surgical Anatomy of the Pectoral Nerves and the Pectoral Musculature. *Clin. Anat.* **2012**, *25*, 559–575. [CrossRef]
32. Creze, M.; Peltier, J.; Havet, E.; Potier, A.; Lefranc, M.; Foulon, P.; Le Gars, D. Anatomy and Surgical Landmarks for the Ansa Pectoralis: Application to Pectoralis Major Nerve Selective Neurotomy. *Surg. Radiol. Anat.* **2012**, *34*, 943–951. [CrossRef] [PubMed]
33. Macchi, V.; Tiengo, C.; Porzionato, A.; Parenti, A.; Stecco, C.; Mazzoleni, F.; De Caro, R. Medial and Lateral Pectoral Nerves: Course and Branches. *Clin. Anat.* **2007**, *20*, 157–162. [CrossRef] [PubMed]

34. Maarrawi, J.; Mertens, P.; Luaute, J.; Vial, C.; Chardonnet, N.; Cosson, M.; Sindou, M. Long-Term Functional Results of Selective Peripheral Neurotomy for the Treatment of Spastic Upper Limb: Prospective Study in 31 Patients. *J. Neurosurg.* **2006**, *104*, 215–225. [CrossRef]
35. Puligopu, A.K.; Purohit, A.K. Outcome of Selective Motor Fasciculotomy in the Treatment of Upper Limb Spasticity. *J. Pediatr. Neurosci.* **2011**, *6*, S118–S125. [CrossRef] [PubMed]
36. Fouad, W. Management of Spastic Hand by Selective Peripheral Neurotomies. *Alex. J. Med.* **2011**, *47*, 201–208. [CrossRef]
37. Mikalef, P.; Power, D. The Role of Neurectomy in the Management of Spasticity of the Upper Limb. *EFORT Open Rev.* **2017**, *2*, 469–473. [CrossRef] [PubMed]
38. Gavilán, J.; Gavilán, C.; Tomás, M.D. Methylene Blue Infusion for Intraoperative Identification of the Parathyroid Glands. *Laryngoscope* **1986**, *96*, 1389–1390. [CrossRef]
39. Aoun, H.D.; Littrup, P.J.; Heath, K.E.; Adam, B.; Prus, M.; Beydoun, R.; Baciewcz, F. Methylene Blue/Collagen Mixture for CT-Guided Presurgical Lung Nodule Marking: High Efficacy and Safety. *J. Vasc. Interv. Radiol.* **2020**, *31*, 1682.e1–1682.e7. [CrossRef]
40. Vegunta, R.K.; Rawlings, A.L.; Jeziorczak, P.M. Methylene Blue: A Simple Marker for Intraoperative Detection of Gastroduodenal Perforations during Laparoscopic Pyloromyotomy. *Surg. Innov.* **2010**, *17*, 11–13. [CrossRef]
41. Bužga, M.; Machytka, E.; Dvořáčková, E.; Švagera, Z.; Stejskal, D.; Máca, J.; Král, J. Methylene Blue: A Controversial Diagnostic Acid and Medication? *Toxicol. Res.* **2022**, *11*, 711–717. [CrossRef]

Journal of
*Personalized Medicine*

MDPI

*Review*

# Image-Guided Musculoskeletal Interventional Radiology in the Personalised Management of Musculoskeletal Tumours

**Hasaam Uldin, Ibrahim Kanbour, Anish Patel and Rajesh Botchu ***

Royal Orthopedic Hospital, Birmingham B31 2AP, UK; hasaam.uldin@nhs.net (H.U.); anish.patel4@nhs.net (A.P.)
* Correspondence: rajesh.botchu@nhs.net

**Abstract:** Musculoskeletal image-guided interventional radiology plays a key role in diagnosing and treating a range of conditions. Recent advances have yielded a wide variety of procedures that can be applied selectively and enable the personalisation of patient care. This review aims to outline the indications, applications, and techniques of subspecialist musculoskeletal oncology interventional procedures that were used at our tertiary referral centre with a focus on how these may be used to personalise patient management. The applications of a range of diagnostic and therapeutic image-guided interventional procedures including different methods of bone and soft tissue sampling, ablation, and augmentation procedures across different types of patients and pathologies are reviewed. To supplement the reviewed literature, we included our own experience and radiology images retrospectively collected from our Picture Archiving and Communication System (PACS). We demonstrate how the range of musculoskeletal image-guided interventions provide flexibility in the diagnosis and management of different tumours across different patient populations. This study provides the musculoskeletal interventional radiologist with insight into how to appropriately utlilise different techniques to optimise the diagnosis, treatment and palliation of tumours.

**Keywords:** radiology; interventional; orthopedics; tertiary care centres; tertiary healthcare; patient care; radiologists; neoplasms

## 1. Introduction

Musculoskeletal oncology is a large and diverse field of growing complexity and scientific development with rapidly emerging medical and surgical developments [1]. Radiology is a key facet of this paradigm shift, in large part thanks to the rapid development of musculoskeletal diagnostic and therapeutic interventional radiology (IR) [2].

Radiology in general has advanced through improvements in radiography, ultrasound, fluoroscopy, Computed Tomography (CT), and Magnetic Resonance Imaging (MRI). These have accelerated the role radiology plays in diagnosis and follow-up of soft tissue and bone tumours. Musculoskeletal IR has more directly benefited from a host of other technological innovations by enabling far more options and flexibility in the options available for minimally invasive procedures.

Musculoskeletal IR entails two main types of procedures. The first are diagnostic procedures, which are used in conjunction with a clinical and radiological assessment to better characterise lesions and subsequently optimise the wider patient management [3,4]. In the context of bone and soft tissue tumours, such procedures predominantly involve biopsy to facilitate a positive diagnosis. Therapeutic options are generally more wide-ranging and we will discuss various types of ablation and augmentation procedures. Treatment aims can be curative or palliative and minimally invasive intervention can play a valuable role in optimising patient care in both types of cases, either alone or in conjunction with other treatments [5].

This review covers the current state of musculoskeletal interventional procedures within the setting of our tertiary tumour centre. The focus is on the principles behind the different techniques used and the flexible application of these to manage a range of conditions.

## 2. Methods

Ultrasound and CT interventional radiology lists at our tertiary orthopaedic oncology centre take place most days of the week. A retrospective search of these lists for procedures performed for oncological indications was carried out using the Radiology Information System (RIS). The indications and techniques of the included procedures were considered. Radiology images were collected from our Picture Archiving and Communication System (PACS).

To support our analysis of the procedures at our centre and contextualise findings within the context of the wider literature, a literature search was carried out in Medline using the terms 'musculoskeletal', 'oncology', 'biopsy', 'intervention', and 'radiology'. The relevant existing literature was reviewed and forms part of the discussion of this review.

## 3. Review and Discussion

### 3.1. General Considerations

Preprocedural planning is perhaps the most crucial aspect of interventional radiology in general and musculoskeletal interventions are no different [3]. Meticulous patient selection, review of existing imaging, and patient preparation are needed before the patient even reaches the interventional radiology department. From our experience, optimisation of these parameters can make even the most difficult procedures proceed smoothly. Conversely, their neglect can be very detrimental and risks complications even in relatively straightforward procedures.

Thorough planning also contextualises any procedures within the wider perspective of patient care. Different patients will have different needs leading to different treatment objectives. Every patient at our institution is, therefore, discussed at a multidisciplinary team (MDT) meeting to ascertain the aims of treatment and thus select the most appropriate procedure, if any. As discussed later in this text, radiological interventions can play a role in both definitive palliative and curative management as well as adjunctly support other treatments such as surgery and medical therapies [5].

Imaging plays a crucial role in narrowing the diagnosis and in selecting patients for biopsy [6]. A wide range of modalities are utilised including radiography, ultrasound, MRI, CT, and nuclear medicine studies. Although many soft tissue and bone lesions are difficult to fully assess on imaging, there are numerous 'do not touch' entities where the imaging characteristics are so clear that a biopsy or intervention would be of no additional benefit and is, therefore, obviated. At our institution, such cases are still discussed with the MDT to gain input from the clinical team before a decision is made not to actively treat.

Imaging also plays an invaluable role in planning percutaneous radiological procedures as well as oncological and surgical treatment [3,6]. The various modalities can help to plan approaches, make equipment choices, and monitor complications. Specific examples of this are discussed below.

### 3.2. Patient Discussion

It is important to remember the patient is at the centre of what is usually a complex care pathway which each clinician must help to navigate. For any musculoskeletal IR procedure, an explanation of the objectives, techniques, and role in overall care must be given at a prior date. This is typically carried out by the oncology team in our institution and forms the first part of the consenting process. On the day of the procedure, the patient meets with the performing interventional radiologist for a detailed discussion on the aims, methods, and risks of the procedure as well as any alternative options, thus completing the consent process. Patients will often raise concerns and queries about technical aspects of the anaesthetic and radiological processes which should be addressed in a comprehensive yet understandable manner.

Most cases at our institution are performed as day cases with patients arriving early in the morning for preprocedural checks and processes. Overnight stays may be necessary for more complex procedures or those with a higher risk of complications.

### 3.3. Procedure Setting

The bulk of intervention work at our institution is performed in a CT scanner room with an ultrasound machine also readily available. Patients are brought from the day case unit into an adjacent waiting recovery area where final preprocedural checks are carried out. Experienced interventional staff including radiographers, nursing, and anaesthetic staff who are familiar with the procedures performed are important to the smooth running and optimisation of patient experience for any procedure.

### 3.4. Diagnostic Procedures

As well as providing diagnostic information in and of itself, imaging is also a means to obtain tissue samples where histopathological analysis is needed for both soft tissue and bony lesions [7]. Several scenarios require such sampling, the most obvious being in cases of clinical and radiological uncertainty as to whether a lesion is benign or malignant. Even where lesions are almost certainly malignant, tissue sampling is usually helpful to identify whether the lesion is a primary tumour or metastasis and detailed histopathological analysis can aid personalisation of subsequent medical oncological care. At our institution, it is only in a few cases that the risk of sampling outweighs any potential palliative or curative benefit from a biopsy.

Most tissue sampling at our institution is carried out under radiological guidance. The main exceptions are very superficial lesions which can be sampled percutaneously without imaging and the minority of lesions which would require en bloc resection regardless of their histological constitution.

#### 3.4.1. Soft Tissue Biopsy

Diagnostic image-guided procedures are a staple of interventional radiology seen in generalist and specialist settings. In the context of musculoskeletal IR, percutaneous core biopsies are the most common procedure. Different approaches are used, mainly dependent on the site, size and composition of the lesion in question.

The easiest lesions to sample are those composed of homogenous soft tissue and located subcutaneously and remote from any important soft tissue structures (e.g., nerves, vessels, tendons, etc.). These can sometimes be biopsied without any imaging whatsoever. However, many lesions will have a degree of heterogeneity or be located within or adjacent to vulnerable structures. These benefit from direct visualisation. Ultrasound is the modality of choice as it provides high-resolution images of superficial structures allowing real-time direct visualisation of the needle as it is placed into the lesion, avoiding adjacent vital structures.

For soft tissue lesions, which are much deeper (e.g., in larger patients or deeper tissues) or more awkward or harder to visualise on ultrasound (e.g., obscured behind bone), CT is an option. While this does not allow real-time visualisation and imparts a radiation dose, visualisation of any area of the body using this generally more completely illustrates the salient anatomy. At our institution, this is carried out by obtaining an initial unenhanced planning helical scan. The skin is then marked and local anaesthetic is administered. Axial slices are then obtained at the site of needle insertion as the local needle is advanced and subsequently exchanged with a biopsy system.

We employ a 'CT fluoroscopy' method to increase accuracy, speed, and patient safety [8]. Unlike the conventional method of entering and exiting the scanner when scanning needle and lesion position, this alternative method consists of staying in the scanning room with the interventional radiologist operating a foot pedal to acquire Partial-Angle CT (PACT) images. Reducing time moving in and out of the scanner means images are acquired quicker thus minimising the dwell time of any needles thereby reducing the risk of inadvertent motion and the need for repeat imaging, ultimately minimising the radiation dose to the patient [9]. However, there is a radiation risk to the operator which must be minimised by ensuring the use of protective lead aprons, thyroid shields, and glasses. The operator's dose is further minimised by limiting the volume of scanning and standing on the detector (rather than the tube) side of the scanner where the dose is minimised [10]. Of course, care should also be taken to only have staff in the room at the time of scanning who must be present, in our institution this is typically only the operating radiologist with an assistant for parts of the procedure where necessary.

For soft tissue biopsies, we employ disposable 14-gauge spring-loaded core biopsy needles (Supercore), typically acquiring four to five samples (Figure 1). In superficial lesions, multiple passes can be made. For deeper lesions, a coaxial system is advised to allow easier biopsy with reduced discomfort and injury.

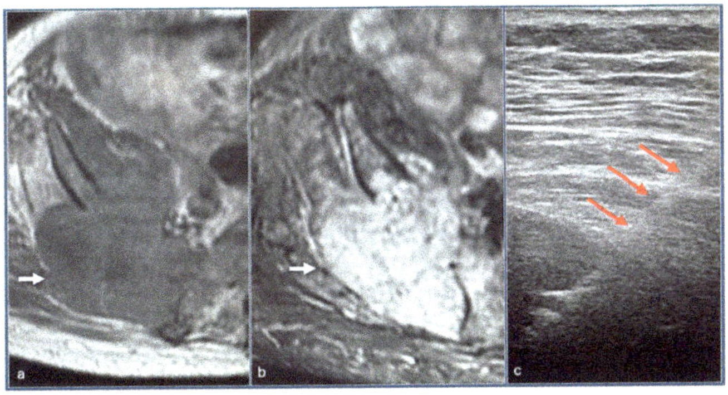


**Figure 1.** Axial T1 (**a**), STIR (**b**) shows tumour (arrow) involving right posterior ilium and Ultrasound-guided biopsy (**c**) showing needle (red arrows).

For all soft tissue and bone lesions apart from those which are immediately subcutaneous, knowledge of the surgical approach is crucial. Although there is some controversy, it is generally accepted that many tumours will seed along the biopsy tract necessitating its resection at the time of any surgery [11,12]. If the biopsy tract is remote to the surgical access, this necessitates widening the surgical field and can limit the extent of treatment as well as reconstruction options. It is, therefore, imperative to agree the biopsy approach with the surgical team prior to the procedure [3]. As a general rule for soft tissue lesions, one must aim not to involve additional compartments to the one involved and to avoid any major neurovascular structures [13].

### 3.4.2. Bone Biopsy

Bone lesion biopsy is a similarly variable process. However, given that such lesions are almost invariably deep and typically have either a calcified component or lie behind a bony cortex, ultrasound is usually not a feasible option. Therefore, CT guidance is the workhorse of these procedures in our centre. As with soft tissue lesions, an initial planning scan is followed by local anaesthetic administration and then 'CT fluoroscopy' imaging as a percutaneous biopsy system is targeted to the lesion.

We use two main needle systems. Most bone lesions can be sampled with a T-Lok eight-gauge system with an inner diamond-tipped stylet and outer cannula. This is inserted through the cortex overlying a bone lesion. Once in the lesion, the stylet is removed and the cannula is advanced to the deep wall of the lesion aiming to trap the core against normal bone on either side. A tray is then inserted through the cannula to acquire the sample. Both tray and cannula are withdrawn together and the sample is then deposited into the relevant histopathology or microbiology pots (Figures 2 and 3). Typically, only one sample is needed unlike in a soft tissue biopsy.

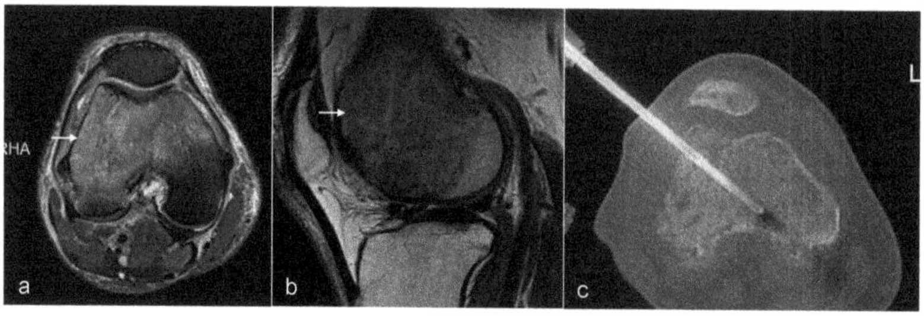

**Figure 2.** Axial T2fat suppressed (**a**), sagittal Proton density (**b**) showing tumour in the distal femur. Axial CT (**c**) showing biopsy needle in the distal femoral lesion.

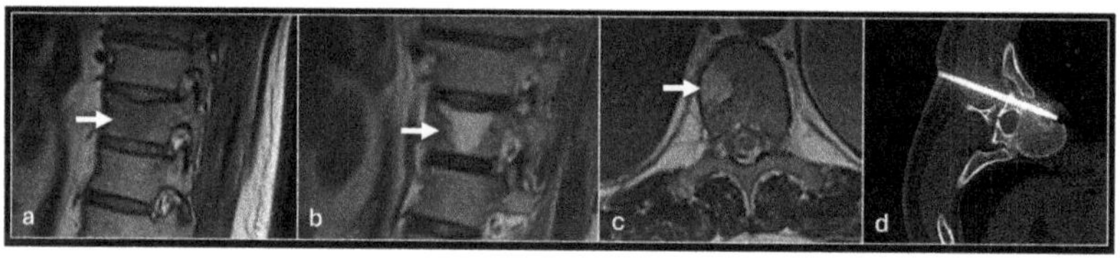

**Figure 3.** Sagittal T1 (**a**), T2 (**b**) and axial T2 (**c**) showing tumour (arrow) in the vertebral body and CT guided biopsy of the lesion (**d**).

While the T-Lok works well for lesions with relatively minimal overlying cortical bone, dense sclerotic bone can be difficult to traverse and requires a drill. Hand and battery-powered drills are available. We employ a Bonopty penetration set which includes a drill. The procedure is similar to with the T-Lok but the drill is inserted after the stylet is removed to penetrate sclerotic bone. The drill itself is taken out at the periphery of the lesion and the cannula is advanced. The radiologist must take care not to destroy the sample itself with the drill, which can easily be inadvertently achieved with small soft lesions within a sclerotic periphery. This is avoided by removing the drill just before entering the lesion itself.

Some bone lesions can consist of large soft-tissue components enclosed within cortical bone. These can be sampled by using a 10 cm × 8 G T-Lok system to gain access through the calcified component. The stylet is then exchanged with a 15 cm × 14 G Supercore biopsy needle (as used in soft tissue biopsy) passed through the cannula (functioning analogously to a coaxial needle) and multiple samples are taken.

Regardless of the type of lesion within the bone, bone biopsies can be technically challenging. A key reason for this is that needle systems are relatively heavy and can be difficult to stabilise under their weight whilst they are in soft tissue but not yet in bone. This can cause the needle to change position when it is released by the radiologist to allow scanning. This is particularly pronounced in the extremities due to the relatively thin, soft tissue and rounded structure. We use several techniques at our institution to adapt to this problem, including stabilisation with steristrips, anchoring against bones, and rolling sterile gauze or towels under the needle [14–16]. Once the needle enters into bone it is generally anchored enough to not move unless it is a particularly long or horizontally orientated needle.

### 3.4.3. Aspiration

Purely cystic lesions—whether in bone or soft tissue—cannot be sampled using biopsy needles alone. Instead, aspiration is used to obtain the material for histopathological and microbiological analysis. Superficial lesions can be sampled with a 21 G 1.5″ 'green' needle under ultrasound guidance. Deeper lesions often require a Quincke-style 22 G needle up to 7″ long. Cystic lesions may be enclosed within the bone and can be accessed using a bone biopsy system with subsequent aspiration through the cannula.

### 3.5. Percutaneous Therapeutic Procedures

Indications for therapeutic musculoskeletal IR procedures fall into two broad categories. Some procedures are performed for definitive treatment, usually of small and isolated lesions that can be targeted and treated percutaneously. These percutaneous therapies have a role as they are minimally invasive and, therefore, generally better tolerated than the surgical alternatives [17,18].

Aside from curative intent, many treatments are carried out for palliative purposes in the context of widespread disease or frailty precluding definitive medical or surgical treatment. As discussed in more detail below, this can include treatment of symptomatic lesions or consolidation of pathological fractures via augmentation procedures. Whilst not ridding the patient of disease, the impact of reduced pain and disability on improving the quality of life achieved through a relatively tolerable procedure can be remarkable.

#### 3.5.1. Ablation

Percutaneous ablation is the destruction of abnormal tissues within bone or soft tissues using needles introduced under image guidance. As with diagnostic procedures, this is a minimally invasive alternative to other options such as surgery. A range of procedures lie under this umbrella but several general principles apply. Regarding indications, ablation can be a curative or adjuvant therapeutic option.

At our institution, ablation is almost always performed with CT guidance which optimises logistical efficiency and procedure planning but some types of ablation can be performed purely under ultrasound, for instance for Morton's Neuroma [19,20]. As for other interventional procedures, imaging is reviewed and a path to the soft tissue is planned. The patient is placed on the scanner in the appropriate position and a radio-opaque grid is applied to the vicinity of the lesion. Following a planning scan, the skin is marked in one or more locations. Local anaesthetic is then administered to subcutaneous tissues. Access to the lesion is usually obtained using either bone or soft tissue biopsy systems (as above) which allows a sample of the lesion to be obtained before ablation. Once the biopsy needle is withdrawn, the cannula remains in situ and an ablation needle is passed through this.

We use two main categories of ablation at our institution—chemical and thermal (see Table 1). The former category largely entails sclerotherapy. From the latter, we mainly apply radiofrequency ablation and cryoablation with other types of energy-based ablation such as microwave, laser, and MRI-guided high-frequency ultrasound rarely used at our institution.

**Table 1.** Table describing the major advantages and disadvantages of different methods of ablation techniques in musculoskeletal IR.

| | Mechanism | Advantages | Disadvantages |
|---|---|---|---|
| **Chemical ablation** | Injection of cytotoxic sclerosant material into a cavity | • Relatively minimal complication rates compared to thermoablation | • Often requieres multiple procedures to complete treatment<br>• Largely limited to treatment of cystic lesions<br>• Sclerosant leakage can cause embolism and tissue necrosis |
| **Radiofrequency Ablation (RFA)** | Delivery of alternating radiofrequency current to induce cytotoxic heat | • Relatively quick<br>• Improved bone consolidation compared to other types of ablation (reduced fracture risk)<br>• Normal cells are relatively resistant to heat shock | • Transient pain is more common and severe<br>• Skin burn which can be severe |

**Table 1.** *Cont.*

| | Mechanism | Advantages | Disadvantages |
|---|---|---|---|
| **Microwave Ablation (MWA)** | Delivery of alternating radiofrequency current to induce heat and cause tumour death | • Fastest at inducing effective coagulation<br>• Can extend deeper with reduced inherent resistance | • Further research needed into optimising parameters |
| **Interstitial Laser Ablation (ILA)** | Laser light- induced heating to causes tumour cell death | • Very precise<br>• Safe and does not require thermoprotection<br>• No risk of skin burn or frostbite | • Limited to benign and small tumours |
| **Cryoablation** | Application of freeze—thaw cycles to induce tumour cell death | • More effective for sclerotic lesions as it can better overcome the thermal insulation properties of cortical bone<br>• Less painful thanks to cryoanalgesia<br>• Cryoadhesional retraction can be used to manipulate the targeted structures<br>• MRI can accurately monitor the cryoablation zone | • Frostbite<br>• Cryoshock<br>• Cryomyositis<br>• Relatively increased bleeding risk compared to heat-based methods as there is no coagulative phase in CA<br>• Limited use in larger tumours (i.e., ≥3 cm or if ≥3 tumours)<br>• Relatively expensive, particularly if using MRI-compatible equipment |
| **High- Frequency Ultrasound (HIFU)** | Cytotoxic heat is generated by focusing ultrasound waves from multiple sources to a common point | • Noninvasive<br>• Relatively safe with minimal risks of burn and inadvertent neurovascular injury | • Can only be used for very superficial lesions in soft tissue or bones with thin cortices<br>• Must be combined with stabilisation if in weight-bearing bones<br>• Works poorly with thermoprotection techniques |

Sclerotherapy

Sclerotherapy is the injection of a sclerosant into a tumour to induce chemical ablation [21]. It is the primary form of chemical ablation for musculoskeletal tumours at our centre. It is mainly used for the treatment of cystic entities—most commonly aneurysmal bone cysts (ABC) but also venous malformations and giant cell tumours (GCTs)—as an alternative to surgical options [22]. It can also be used as an adjuvant treatment for locally aggressive GCTs and cystic malignant tumours but surgery en bloc remains the treatment of choice for these lesions.

A wide range of injectants are used including polidocanol, ethanol, and warm Ringer's lactate (Hartmann's) solution [13,15–17,23,24]. At our centre and others, doxycycline is agitated with an equal volume of air and used for injection [25]. This antibiotic has shown safety and efficacy in suppressing tumour growth and stimulating bone formation, thus rendering it a useful agent for sclerotherapy in both appendicular and axial lesions [14,18,19,25–27].

The cyst is typically accessed using an 11 G bone biopsy needle. If the lesion is multiloculated, the needle is agitated to break up the septations to facilitate communication and its contents are aspirated. The position is confirmed with the injection of iodinated contrast which also has the benefit of confirming no intravascular communication or leak into other adjacent structures is present as also described in the existing literature [28,29]. If the lesion cannot be completely opacified, further punctures may be required. Once satisfactorily opacified, the sclerosant is injected and subsequently aspirated to minimise the risk of leakage. This allows the lesion to consolidate or involute over successive procedures (Figures 4 and 5).

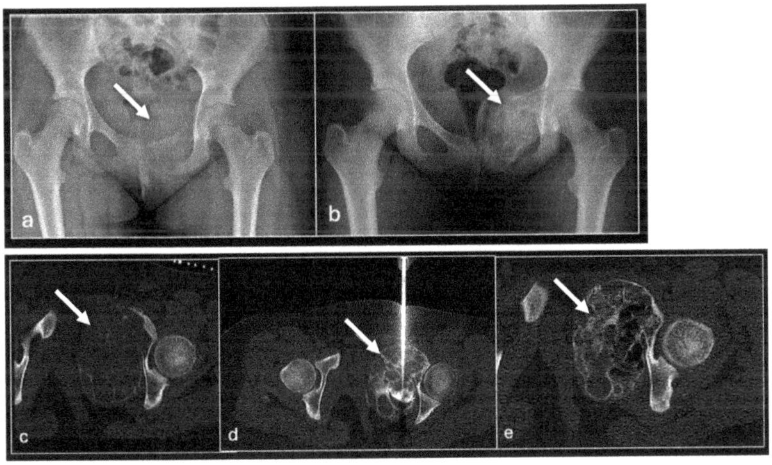

**Figure 4.** AP radiograph of pelvis (**a**) showing destructive lesion of left pubis and superior pubic ramus (arrow) with marked consolidation post three sessions of sclerotherapy (**b**). Axial CT imaging pre sclerotherapy (c), intraprocedural (**d**), and following three sessions of sclerotherapy (**e**) to the lesion (arrow).

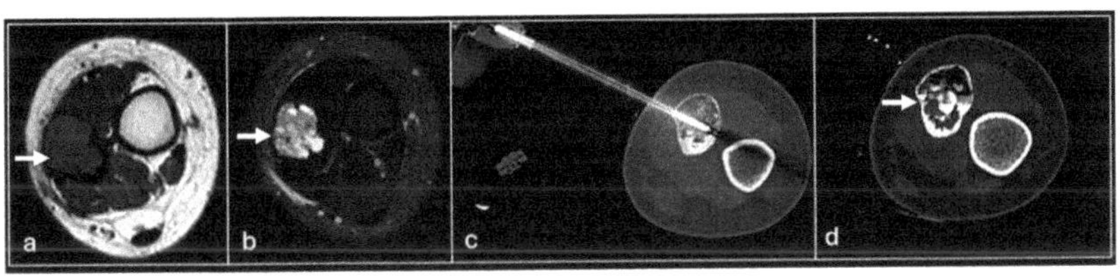

**Figure 5.** Axial T1 (**a**), STIR (**b**) showing aneurysmal bone cyst of fibula (arrow) treated with sclerotherapy under CT guidance (**c**,**d**).

Sclerotherapy advantageously does not suffer from the risks to adjacent tissues and skin seen with the thermoablation techniques described above. Complication rates are low but sclerosant leakage or injection into vascular structures is a potential risk which can lead to embolism and tissue necrosis. Perhaps the biggest drawback is that repeat procedures are frequently necessary, particularly for larger lesions resulting in substantial time and resource allocation [30–32].

Thermoablation

In thermoablation, the aim is to rapidly change cell temperature to induce necrosis or coagulation in tumour cells while preserving the adjacent normal cells, the latter of which are typically more resistant to temperature change [33]. The ablated area then involutes and is replaced with soft tissue or bone over subsequent weeks to months. Augmentation procedures (see below) can be used in larger ablated areas to maintain structural integrity during the healing process [34].

Radiofrequency ablation (RFA), microwave ablation (MWA), interstitial laser ablation (ILA), and high-frequency ultrasound (HIFU) all apply ablative heat energy in different ways. Cryoablation instead uses ice balls to destroy tissue.

- Radiofrequency Ablation

Radiofrequency ablation has been used for over a century in a range of non-musculoskeletal and non-oncological settings [35,36]. Its application to tumour ablation has increased in recent years. There are several types, with our institution using pulsed RFA.

This technique is particularly used as a first-line curative option in osteoid osteomas and osteoblastomas. It is also effective in the cure of chondroblastoma [37,38]. As a palliative option, it has been used for painful bony and soft tissue metastases as well as myeloma and can be combined with cement augmentation to restore function [36,39,40].

Radiofrequency ablation uses temperatures of up to 95 °C applied over several minutes to induce tumour cell coagulation necrosis. Technically, this is achieved by positioning an RFA needle (the cathode) into the lesion using a similar approach to a bone biopsy (i.e., with a coaxial biopsy needle system including a drill) and applying a grounding pad to the patient's thigh (the anode). Most treated lesions are surrounded by cortical bone, thus insulating adjacent structures from the hot needle tip and effectively heating the tumour. Before introducing the RFA needle, a biopsy is typically taken to confirm the suspected diagnosis.

As well as bearing in mind the 'standard' complications associated with percutaneous procedures involving bone such as fracture, infection, pain, and injury to neurovascular structures, RFA also can cause thermal injuries perilesional soft tissue as well as significant skin burns at the needle and grounding pad sites. Techniques such as injection of fluid or $CO_2$ to separate structures or thermal monitoring of adjacent tissues can minimise the risk of injury (Figures 6–11).

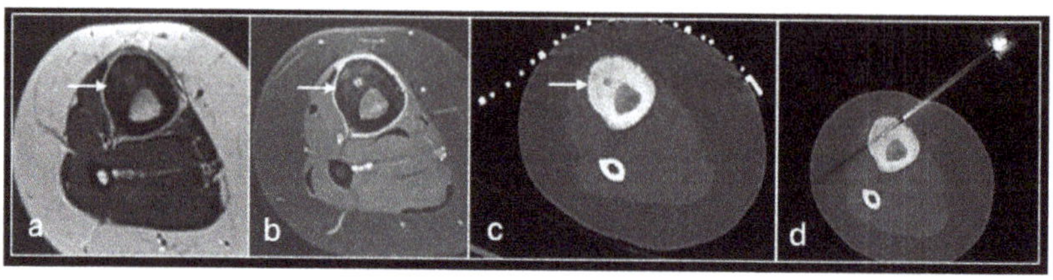

**Figure 6.** Axial T1 (**a**), STIR (**b**), CT (**c**) showing osteoid osteoma of tibia (arrow) treated with radiofrequency ablation (**d**).

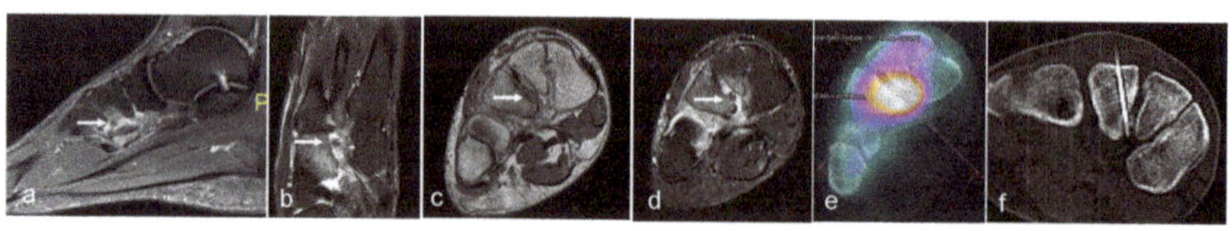

**Figure 7.** Sagittal (**a**) and axial (**b**) T2 fat-suppressed, coronal PD (**c**) and PD fat-saturated (**d**), SPECT CT (**e**) all showing osteoid osteoma of the lateral cuneiform (white arrows) treated with radiofrequency ablation (**f**).

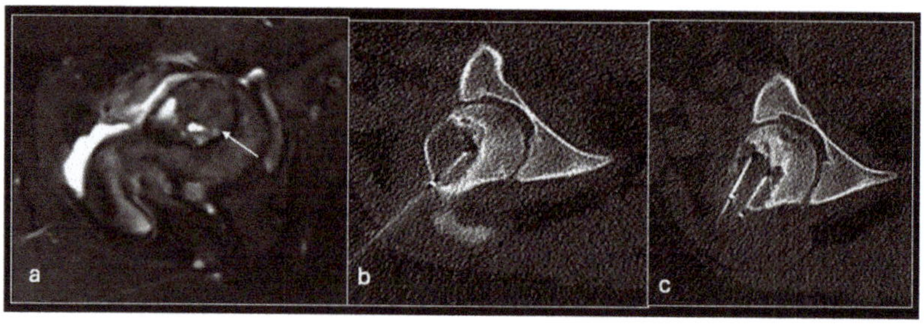

**Figure 8.** Axial STIR (**a**) showing femoral head chondroblastoma (arrow) treated with CT-guided radiofrequency ablation with multiple needles (**b**,**c**).

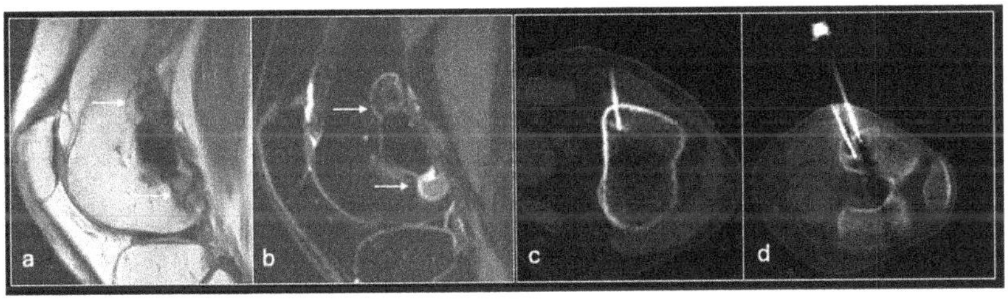


**Figure 9.** Sagittal T1 (**a**), STIR (**b**) showing recurrence of GCT cranial and caudal (arrows) to prior cementation subsequently treated with radiofrequency ablation (**c**,**d**).

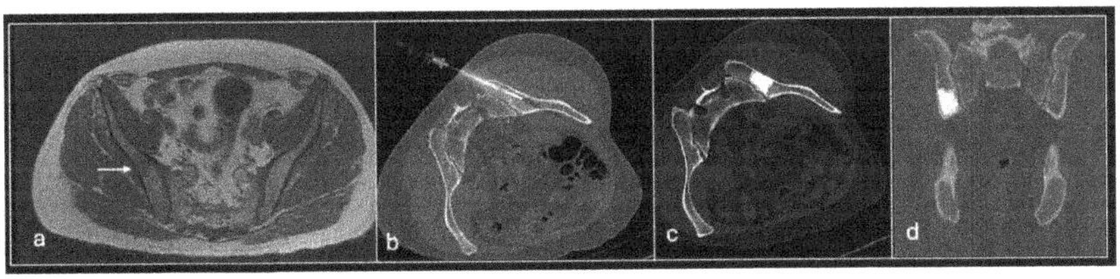


**Figure 10.** Axial T1 (**a**) showing metastasis in right ilium (arrow) (**b**) treated with radiofrequency ablation. Post-cementoplasty axial (**c**) and coronal (**d**) CT post-cementoplasty.

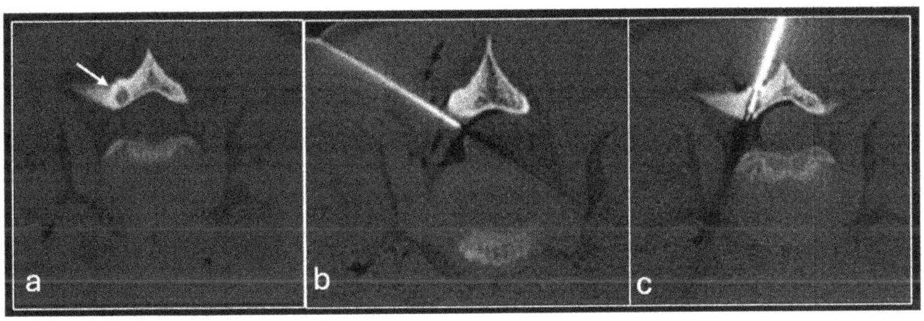


**Figure 11.** Axial CT showing osteoid osteoma of lumbar spine (arrow) (**a**) treated with radiofrequency ablation with neuroprotection using air (**b**,**c**).

- Microwave Ablation

Microwave ablation (MWA) is another heat-based method whereby antennae are inserted into the tumour and an electromagnetic field is used to generate the heat. The advantages to this method over RFA include faster induction of coagulation necrosis, reduced heat loss, and less variably inherent resistance [41,42]. These features allow deeper extension and a larger ablation zone. Like RFA, MWA risks burning the ablation site but does not use a grounding pad and, therefore, does not result in skin burns here [43].

In the liver, MWA shows a more consistent and faster response than RFA and allows the use of multiple probes. These factors favour its suitability for larger tumours and those in close proximity to neurovascular structures [44]. The literature delineating the role of MWA in musculoskeletal tumour treatment is relatively sparse but several successful series have found MWA is an effective curative option for osteoid osteomas, perhaps superior to RFA [41,43].

- Laser Ablation

Laser ablation is also known as Interstitial Laser Ablation (ILA) or Laser Interstitial Thermal Therapy (LITT). The underpinning principle is the delivery of infrared light through optical fibres to generate head and induce coagulation necrosis [45]. This is a relatively new method first reported in 1997 but key potential benefits over MWA and RFA are more precise and predictable energy delivery into the lesion as well as MRI compatibility [46,47]. Efficacy was demonstrated in small benign tumours (such as osteoid osteomas and vascular malformations) as well as malignant tumours outside of bone but no clinical applications for malignant lesions are present in the existing literature [48,49].

- Cryoablation

Cryoablation is the direct rapid cooling of lesions to temperatures as low as −100 °C to induce crystallisation of intracellular water thus causing apoptosis. This is achieved using rapidly expanding gas (usually argon) to cause a rapid drop in temperature via a phenomenon termed the Joule–Thompson effect [50]. Multiple freeze–thaw cycles are usually required with the latter achieved using helium gas infusion (Figure 12).

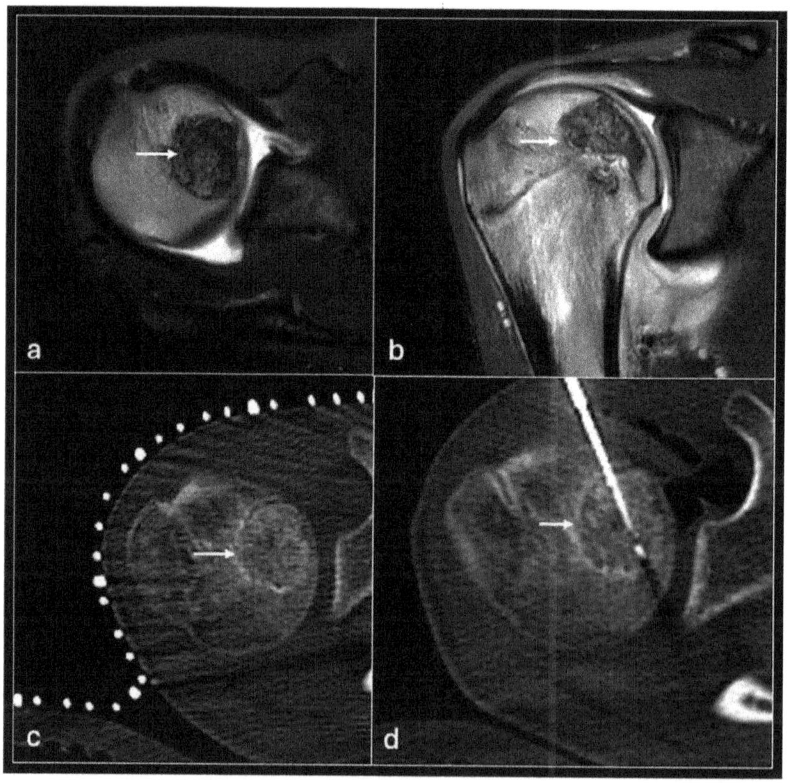


**Figure 12.** STIR axial (**a**), coronal (**b**) showing chondroblastoma in the humeral head (arrow) treated with CT-guided cryotherapy (**c**,**d**).

Indications are more wide-ranging than other forms of ablation. Curative oncological indications include benign desmoid tumours, osteoid osteomas, vascular malformations, aneurysmal bone cysts and neuromas [50,51]. Malignant lesions such as bone metastases can be treated curatively but palliation of painful bone metastases is a more established process [52–54].

Like other thermoablation methods, cryoablation is achieved by percutaneously inserting probes into the lesion. Unlike RFA, multiple needles can be used allowing more flexibility in tumours of different geometry and coverage of a larger ablation area. However, the ablation process takes longer and is more expensive than other options. As well as general thermoablation risks to the skin and perilesional structures, specific risks include cryomyositis (peritumoural muscle inflammation) and cryoshock (a systemic inflammatory response from the release of inflammatory mediators). Numerous methods can be employed to minimise inadvertent freezing risk such as hydrodissection and active or passive warming of the adjacent structures [33,55]. Temperature monitoring and direct visualisation of the ice ball using CT or ultrasound during cryotherapy can also reduce the risk of injuring adjacent structures [56,57].

- High-Frequency Ultrasound

Magnetic Resonance-Guided High-Intensity Focused Ultrasound (MRg-HIFU) is the non-invasive focusing of ultrasound onto a lesion to induce heat and coagulation necrosis within the lesion. Musculoskeletal applications include osteoid osteoma/osteoblastoma and bone metastases (particularly for pain relief) but clinical utility specifically in the cure of musculoskeletal tumours remains relatively sparse [58–60].

The key benefit of percutaneous ablation is reduced complications from the non-invasive nature such as a much lower risk of fracture or infection. However, efficacy is limited to relatively small superficial structures within thin, flat bones and away from any perilesional vital structures [58,60].

### 3.5.2. Cement Augmentation

Cement augmentation is the injection of polymethylmethacrylate cement (PMMA) mixture into a bony defect to restore bony structural integrity and provide pain relief. The most common form is vertebroplasty in the context of vertebral compression fractures which—in the setting of oncology—include pathological fractures with underlying myeloma or metastases with resultant pain and disability refractory to conservative treatment. The procedure is also a useful adjunct following percutaneous ablation to restore structural integrity following bone destruction, particularly for larger lesions [33] (Figures 13 and 14).

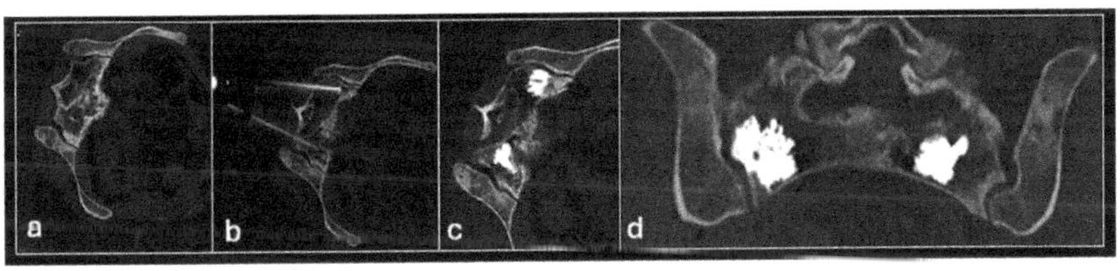


**Figure 13.** Axial CT (**a**) showing metastasis in the sacrum. Images (**b**–**d**) showing sacroplasty with cement in both sacral ala.

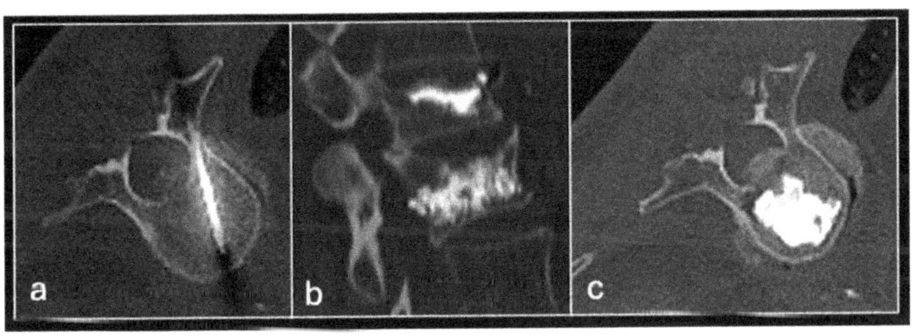


**Figure 14.** CT-guided vertebroplasty showing needle in the vertebral body (**a**) and sagittal (**b**) and axial (**c**) showing cement within the vertebral bodies.

A relatively novel procedure described in the literature combines Ablation, Osteoplasty, Reinforcement, and Internal Fixation (AORIF) and it has been applied most commonly in the pelvis and proximal femora [60–62]. This is performed by introducing cannulated screws into osteolytic lesions as portals for ablation, balloon osteoplasty, and the delivery of bone cement to facilitate the treatment of these lesions.

The most common type of cement augmentation at our centre is vertebroplasty. This is typically performed via a transpedicular approach into the lesion using an 11 G or 14 G bone biopsy needle system. Biopsy samples may be taken with the PMMA and then injected into the defect. A modified procedure is the kyphoplasty in which cement injection is preceded by the inflation of a balloon device in the vertebral body to create space with the cavity then filled with the cement. This is more effective in pain relief and minimises leakage but results in a longer and more expensive procedure [4,63].

Other variants with similar underlying principles include sacroplasty and acetabuloplasty. Complications to be aware of include cement leakage, which can lead to cement thrombosis, pulmonary emboli and compression of adjacent structures [64,65]. Nevertheless, cement augmentation generally remains a relatively safe and effective minimally invasive procedure, which can greatly improve patient quality of life in a palliative setting.

## 4. Conclusions

Advancements in musculoskeletal interventional radiology have yielded a wide range of diagnostic and therapeutic minimally invasive procedures. We illustrated how these have introduced more flexibility to the management of soft tissue and bone tumours and provide alternatives to more traditional surgical and oncological approaches in curative and palliative settings.

It is virtually certain that the continued development of minimally invasive tissue sampling, ablation, and augmentation procedures amongst others will add to the arsenal of treatment options across a range of clinical oncological applications. This study has provided the reader with insight into how these techniques and principles can be applied to different clinical scenarios to optimise patient management.

**Author Contributions:** Conceptualisation, H.U. and R.B.; methodology, H.U. and R.B.; formal analysis, H.U. and R.B.; resources, H.U. and R.B.; writing—original draft preparation, H.U., R.B., I.K. and A.P.; writing—review and editing, R.B.; supervision, H.U.; project administration, R.B. All authors have read and agreed to the published version of the manuscript.

**Funding:** This research received no external funding.

**Institutional Review Board Statement:** Not applicable.

**Informed Consent Statement:** Not applicable.

**Data Availability Statement:** No new data were created or analysed in this study. Data sharing is not applicable to this article.

**Conflicts of Interest:** The authors declare no conflict of interest.

## References

1. Bergovec, M.; Kubat, O.; Smerdelj, M.; Seiwerth, S.; Bonevski, A.; Orlic, D. Epidemiology of musculoskeletal tumors in a national referral orthopedic department. A study of 3482 cases. *Cancer Epidemiol.* **2015**, *39*, 298–302. [CrossRef] [PubMed]
2. Recht, M.P.; White, L.M.; Fritz, J.; Resnick, D.L. Advances in Musculoskeletal Imaging: Recent Developments and Predictions for the Future. *Radiology* **2023**, *308*, e230615. [CrossRef] [PubMed]
3. Meek, R.D.; Mills, M.K.; Hanrahan, C.J.; Beckett, B.R.; Leake, R.L.; Allen, H.; Williams, D.D.; Tommack, M.; Schmahmann, S.; Hansford, B.G. Pearls and Pitfalls for Soft-Tissue and Bone Biopsies: A Cross-Institutional Review. *Radiographics* **2020**, *40*, 266–290. [CrossRef] [PubMed]
4. Bansal, A.; Goyal, A.; Gamanagatti, S.; Srivastava, D.N.; Manhas, V. Current updates in image-guided musculoskeletal interventions. *J. Clin. Orthop. Trauma* **2021**, *22*, 101601. [CrossRef] [PubMed]
5. Bădilă, A.E.; Rădulescu, D.M.; Niculescu, A.-G.; Grumezescu, A.M.; Rădulescu, M.; Rădulescu, A.R. Recent Advances in the Treatment of Bone Metastases and Primary Bone Tumors: An Up-to-Date Review. *Cancers* **2021**, *13*, 4229. [CrossRef] [PubMed]
6. Isaac, A.; Dalili, D.; Dalili, D.; Weber, M.-A. State-of-the-art imaging for diagnosis of metastatic bone disease. *Radiologe* **2020**, *60* (Suppl. S1), 1–16. [CrossRef] [PubMed]

7. Exner, G.U.; Kurrer, M.O.; Mamisch-Saupe, N.; Cannon, S.R. The Tactics and Technique of Musculoskeletal Biopsy. 23 February 2017. Available online: https://eor.bioscientifica.com/view/journals/eor/2/2/2058-5241.2.160065.xml (accessed on 14 December 2024).
8. Fu, Y.F.; Li, C.C.; Cao, W.; Wang, T.; Shi, Y.B. Computed Tomography Fluoroscopy–Guided Versus Conventional Computed Tomography–Guided Lung Biopsy: A Systematic Review and Meta-analysis. *J. Comput. Assist. Tomogr.* **2020**, *44*, 571–577. [CrossRef]
9. Cahalane, A.M.; Habibollahi, S.; Staffa, S.J.; Yang, K.; Fintelmann, F.J.; Chang, C.Y. Helical CT versus intermittent CT fluoroscopic guidance for musculoskeletal needle biopsies: Impact on radiation exposure, procedure time, diagnostic yield, and adverse events. *Skelet. Radiol.* **2023**, *52*, 1119–1126. [CrossRef]
10. Knott, E.A.; Rose, S.D.; Wagner, M.G.; Lee, F.T.; Radtke, J.; Anderson, D.R.; Zlevor, A.M.; Lubner, M.G.; Hinshaw, J.L.; Szczykutowicz, T.P. CT Fluoroscopy for Image-Guided Procedures: Physician Radiation Dose During Full-Rotation and Partial-Angle CT Scanning. *J. Vasc. Interv. Radiol.* **2021**, *32*, 439–446. [CrossRef] [PubMed]
11. Lai, C.; Long, J.R.; Larsen, B.T.; Iturregui, J.M.; Wilke, B.K.; Goulding, K.A. Percutaneous biopsy of musculoskeletal tumors and the potential for needle tract seeding: Technical considerations, current controversies, and outcomes. *Skelet. Radiol.* **2023**, *52*, 505–516. [CrossRef]
12. Seeger, L.L. Revisiting tract seeding and compartmental anatomy for percutaneous image-guided musculoskeletal biopsies. *Skelet. Radiol.* **2019**, *48*, 499–501. [CrossRef]
13. Mavrogenis, A.F.; Altsitzioglou, P.; Tsukamoto, S.; Errani, C. Biopsy Techniques for Musculoskeletal Tumors: Basic Principles and Specialized Techniques. *Curr. Oncol.* **2024**, *31*, 900–917. [CrossRef] [PubMed]
14. Espinosa, L.A.; Jamadar, D.A.; Jacobson, J.A.; DeMaeseneer, M.O.; Ebrahim, F.S.; Sabb, B.J.; Kretschmer, M.T.; Biermann, J.S.; Kim, S.-M. CT-Guided Biopsy of Bone: A Radiologist's Perspective. *Am. J. Roentgenol.* **2008**, *190*, W283–W289. [CrossRef] [PubMed]
15. McLoughlin, E.; Iqbal, A.; Patel, A.; James, S.L.; Botchu, R. Dual steristrip technique: A novel use of steristrips to reduce operator radiation dose during CT-guided intervention. *Skelet. Radiol.* **2019**, *48*, 1617–1620. [CrossRef] [PubMed]
16. Botchu, R.; Nischal, N.; Botchu, B.; Iyengar, K.P. Piggyback Technique—A Safe Way of Performing Rib Biopsy. *Indian J. Radiol. Imaging* **2023**, *33*, 541–542. [CrossRef] [PubMed]
17. Parvinian, A.; Welch, B.T.; Callstrom, M.R.; Kurup, A.N. Trends in Musculoskeletal Ablation: Emerging Indications and Techniques. *Tech. Vasc. Interv. Radiol.* **2020**, *23*, 100678. [CrossRef] [PubMed]
18. Tomasian, A.; Filippiadis, D.K.; Tutton, S.; Deschamps, F.; Cazzato, R.L.; Prologo, J.D.; Kelekis, A.; Levy, J.; Gangi, A.; Garnon, J.; et al. Comprehensive Palliative Musculoskeletal Interventional Radiology Care for Patients with Cancer. *Radiographics* **2022**, *42*, 1654–1669. [CrossRef]
19. Llombart, R.; Mariscal, G.; Benlloch, M.; Barrios, C.; Llombart-Ais, R. Systematic Review and Meta-Analysis of Radiofrequency Ablation for Morton's Neuroma: Outcomes and Predictors of Success. *Am. J. Phys. Med. Rehabil.* **2024**. [CrossRef] [PubMed]
20. Koltsakis, E.; Klontzas, M.E.; Kakkos, G.A.; Karantanas, A.H. Ultrasound-guided treatment of Morton's neuroma. *J. Ultrason.* **2021**, *21*, E134–E138. [CrossRef] [PubMed]
21. Weber, K.S.; Jensen, C.L.; Petersen, M.M. Sclerotherapy as a primary or salvage procedure for aneurysmal bone cysts: A single-center experience. *World J. Orthop.* **2023**, *14*, 698–706. [CrossRef]
22. Wong, M.N.; Braswell, L.E.; Murakami, J.W. Doxycycline sclerotherapy of cervical spine aneurysmal bone cysts: Single-institution 13-year experience. *Pediatr. Radiol.* **2022**, *52*, 1528–1538. [CrossRef] [PubMed]
23. Waikakul, S.; Asavamongkolkul, A.; Phimolsarnti, R. Use of warm Ringer's lactate solution in the management of locally advanced giant cell tumor of bone. *Int. J. Clin. Oncol.* **2016**, *21*, 177–185. [CrossRef]
24. Aristiyadi, K.E.B.; Hadar, A.K.; Usman, H.A.; Wienanda, A.K.; Nugraha, H.G.; Hilman. Sclerotherapy with absolute alcohol in a child with spinal aneurysmal bone cyst: A case report. *Radiol. Case Rep.* **2024**, *19*, 4854–4860. [CrossRef]
25. Foo, M.I.; Nicol, K.; Murakami, J.W. Skull base chondroblastoma with aneurysmal bone cyst–like changes treated with percutaneous radiofrequency ablation and doxycycline sclerotherapy: Illustrative case. *J. Neurosurg. Case Lessons* **2022**, *4*, CASE22436. [CrossRef]
26. Wong, M.N.B.; Murakami, J.W. Doxycycline Sclerotherapy of Mandibular Aneurysmal Bone Cysts: A Brief Clinical Study. *J. Craniofacial Surg.* **2024**, 10–1097. [CrossRef]
27. Wong, M.N.; Begley, K.A.; Braswell, L.E.; Alexander, J.H.; Lillis, A.P.; Smetzer, S.M.; Murakami, J.W. Doxycycline Sclerotherapy of Aneurysmal and Unicameral Bone Cysts in the Appendicular Skeleton and Pelvis: Single-Center 14-Year Experience. *J. Vasc. Interv. Radiol.* **2024**, *35*, 1785–1792.e5. [CrossRef] [PubMed]
28. Moussa, A.M.; Aly, A.K.; Maybody, M.; Camacho, J.C., Ridouani, F.; Gonzalez-Aguirre, A.J.; Santos, E. A comparison of lymphatic embolization and sclerotherapy in the management of iatrogenic abdominopelvic lymphoceles following oncological surgery. *Diagn. Interv. Radiol.* **2023**, *29*, 542–547. [CrossRef]
29. Dalili, D.; Parker, J.; Mirzaian, A.; Teh, J.; Bratby, M.; Mansour, R.; Reynolds, J. Aneurysmal bone cysts in the spine, causing neurological compromise: Safety and clinical efficacy of sclerotherapy utilizing sodium Tetradecyl sulfate foam. *Skelet. Radiol.* **2021**, *50*, 2433–2447. [CrossRef]
30. Hegde, G.; Iyengar, K.P.; Kurisunkal, V.; Sharma, G.K.; Ariyaratne, S.; Botchu, R. Current role and future applications of image-guided interventional procedures in musculoskeletal oncology—A narrative review. *J. Orthop.* **2023**, *44*, 99–106. [CrossRef]

31. Jasper, J.; van der Heijden, L.; van Rijswijk, C.S.P.; van de Sande, M.A.J. Efficacy of Sclerotherapy with Polidocanol (Ethoxysclerol) in Primary Aneurysmal Bone Cysts in Children and Adolescents. *J. Pediatr. Orthop.* **2021**, *41*, e555. [CrossRef]
32. Kumar, D.; Kumar, S.; Kumar, D.; Patel, B.M.; Kumar, A.; Kumar, S.; Waliullah, S. Sclerotherapy for Aneurysmal Bone Cyst: A Single-Center Experience. *Cureus* **2021**, *13*, e18469. [CrossRef] [PubMed]
33. Dalili, D.; Isaac, A.; Bazzocchi, A.; Åström, G.; Bergh, J.; Lalam, R.; Weber, M.-A.; Fritz, J.; Mansour, R. Interventional Techniques for Bone and Musculoskeletal Soft Tissue Tumors: Current Practices and Future Directions—Part I. Ablation. *Semin. Musculoskelet. Radiol.* **2020**, *24*, 692–709. [CrossRef]
34. Palussière, J.; Pellerin-Guignard, A.; Descat, E.; Cornélis, F.; Dixmérias, F. Radiofrequency ablation of bone tumours. *Diagn. Interv. Imaging* **2012**, *93*, 660–664. [CrossRef] [PubMed]
35. Tseng, H.; Lin, S.-E.; Chang, Y.-L.; Chen, M.-H.; Hung, S.-H. Determining the critical effective temperature and heat dispersal pattern in monopolar radiofrequency ablation using temperature-time integration. *Exp. Ther. Med.* **2015**, *11*, 763–768. [CrossRef] [PubMed]
36. Strand, N.H.; Hagedorn, J.M.; Dunn, T.; Johnson, B.; Abd-Elsayed, A.; Covington, S.; Freeman, J.; Dawodu, A.; Maloney, J. Advances in radiofrequency ablation: Mechanism of action and technology. *Ann. Palliat. Med.* **2024**, *13*, 1028–1034. [CrossRef]
37. Kulkarni, S.S.; Shetty, N.S.; Gala, K.B.; Shariq, M.; Gulia, A.; Polnaya, A.M.; Shetty, N.G.; Janu, A.K.; Choudhari, A.; Puri, A. Percutaneous Radiofrequency Ablation of Appendicular Skeleton Chondroblastoma—An Experience from a Tertiary Care Cancer Center. *J. Vasc. Interv. Radiol.* **2021**, *32*, 504–509. [CrossRef]
38. Sulaiman, S.R.K.; Al-Zubaidi, S.A.M.; Sakrana, A.A. Radio Frequency Ablation for the Treatment of Appendicular Skeleton Chondroblastoma: Is It an Excellent Alternative? Systematic Review and Meta-Analysis. *Indian J. Radiol. Imaging* **2022**, *32*, 523–530. [CrossRef] [PubMed]
39. Cazzato, R.L.; Garnon, J.; Koch, G.; Dalili, D.; Rao, P.P.; Weiss, J.; Bauones, S.; Auloge, P.; de Marini, P.; Gangi, A. Musculoskeletal interventional oncology: Current and future practices. *Br. J. Radiol.* **2020**, *93*, 20200465. [CrossRef]
40. Faiella, E.; Vaccarino, F.; Pacella, G.; Santucci, D.; Vergantino, E.; Bruno, A.; Ragone, R.; Zobel, B.B.; Grasso, R.F. Exploring the Efficacy of Combining Radiofrequency Thermal Ablation or Microwave Ablation with Vertebroplasty for Pain Control and Disease Management in Metastatic Bone Disease—A Systematic Review. *Curr. Oncol.* **2024**, *31*, 5422–5438. [CrossRef]
41. Parisot, L.; Grillet, F.; Verdot, P.; Danner, A.; Brumpt, E.; Aubry, S. CT-guided microwave ablation of osteoid osteoma: Long-term outcome in 28 patients. *Diagn. Interv. Imaging* **2022**, *103*, 427–432. [CrossRef]
42. Sgalambro, F.; Zugaro, L.; Bruno, F.; Palumbo, P.; Salducca, N.; Zoccali, C.; Barile, A.; Masciocchi, C.; Arrigoni, F. Interventional Radiology in the Management of Metastases and Bone Tumors. *J. Clin. Med.* **2022**, *11*, 3265. [CrossRef] [PubMed]
43. Westlake, B.; Mazzi, J.; Tedesco, N. Osteoid Osteoma Treatment with Microwave Ablation: A Report of Two Cases. *Medicina* **2021**, *57*, 470. [CrossRef]
44. Izzo, F.; Granata, V.; Grassi, R.; Fusco, R.; Palaia, R.; Delrio, P.; Carrafiello, G.; Azoulay, D.; Petrillo, A.; A Curley, S. Radiofrequency Ablation and Microwave Ablation in Liver Tumors: An Update. *Oncol.* **2019**, *24*, e990–e1005. [CrossRef] [PubMed]
45. Ryan, A.; Byrne, C.; Pusceddu, C.; Buy, X.; Tsoumakidou, G.; Filippiadis, D. CIRSE Standards of Practice on Thermal Ablation of Bone Tumours. *Cardiovasc. Interv. Radiol.* **2022**, *45*, 591–605. [CrossRef] [PubMed]
46. Foster, R.C.; Stavas, J.M. Bone and Soft Tissue Ablation. *Semin. Interv. Radiol.* **2014**, *31*, 167. [CrossRef]
47. Gangi, A.; Dietemann, J.L.; Gasser, B.; Mortazavi, R.; Brunner, P.; Mourou, M.Y.; Dosch, J.C.; Durckel, J.; Marescaux, J.; Roy, C. Interstitial laser photocoagulation of osteoid osteomas with use of CT guidance. *Radiology* **1997**, *203*, 843–848. [CrossRef]
48. Hernández-Porras, B.C.; Plancarte, R.; Andrade, J.M.; Koyyalagunta, D. Bone cancer pain. *Indian J. Pain* **2021**, *35*, 4. [CrossRef]
49. Geoghegan, R.; Zhang, L.; Priester, A.M.; Wu, H.H.; Marks, L.; Natarajan, S. Interstitial Optical Monitoring of Focal Laser Ablation. *IEEE Trans. Biomed. Eng.* **2022**, *69*, 2545–2556. [CrossRef] [PubMed]
50. Papalexis, N.; Savarese, L.G.; Peta, G.; Errani, C.; Tuzzato, G.; Spinnato, P.; Ponti, F.; Miceli, M.; Facchini, G. The New Ice Age of Musculoskeletal Intervention: Role of Percutaneous Cryoablation in Bone and Soft Tissue Tumors. *Curr. Oncol.* **2023**, *30*, 6744–6770. [CrossRef]
51. Bodard, S.; Geevarghese, R.; Razakamanantsoa, L.; Frandon, J.; Petre, E.N.; Marcelin, C.; Cornelis, F.H. Percutaneous cryoablation in soft tissue tumor management: An educational review. *Insights Imaging* **2024**, *15*, 278. [CrossRef]
52. Autrusseau, P.-A.; Cazzato, R.; De Marini, P.; Auloge, P.; Koch, G.; Dalili, D.; Weiss, J.; Mayer, T.; Garnon, J.; Gangi, A. Pain relief and local tumour control following percutaneous image-guided cryoablation for spine metastasis: A 12-year single-centre experience. *Clin. Radiol.* **2021**, *76*, 674–680. [CrossRef] [PubMed]
53. Khanmohammadi, S.; Noroozi, A.; Yekaninejad, M.S.; Rezaei, N. Cryoablation for the Palliation of Painful Bone Metastasis: A Systematic Review. *Cardiovasc. Interv. Radiol.* **2023**, *46*, 1469–1482. [CrossRef] [PubMed]
54. Kita, K.; Nakamura, T.; Yamanaka, T.; Yoshida, K.; Hagi, T.; Asanuma, K.; Nakatsuka, A.; Sudo, A. Successful treatment with cryoablation in a patient with bone metastasis in the mid-shaft femur: A case report. *OncoTargets Ther.* **2019**, *12*, 2949–2953. [CrossRef]
55. Chen, C.; Garlich, J.; Vincent, K.; Brien, E. Postoperative complications with cryotherapy in bone tumors. *J. Bone Oncol.* **2017**, *7*, 13–17. [CrossRef]
56. Schreuder, H.W.; van Egmond, J.; van Beem, H.B.; Veth, R.P. Monitoring during cryosurgery of bone tumors. *J. Surg. Oncol.* **1997**, *65*, 40–45. [CrossRef]

57. Al-Assam, H.; Botchu, R.; Azzopardi, C.; Stevenson, J.D.; James, S.L.; Patel, A. Measurement Analysis of Ice Ball Size during CT-Guided Cryoablation Procedures for Better Prediction of Final Ice Ball Size and Avoidance of Complications. *Indian J. Radiol. Imaging* **2023**, *33*, 321–326. [CrossRef]
58. Bing, F.; Garnon, J.; Tsoumakidou, G.; Enescu, I.; Ramamurthy, N.; Gangi, A. Imaging-guided percutaneous cryotherapy of bone and soft-tissue tumors: What is the impact on the muscles around the ablation site? *AJR Am. J. Roentgenol.* **2014**, *202*, 1361–1365. [CrossRef]
59. Bing, F.; Vappou, J.; de Mathelin, M.; Gangi, A. Targetability of osteoid osteomas and bone metastases by MR-guided high intensity focused ultrasound (MRgHIFU). *Int. J. Hyperth.* **2018**, *35*, 471–479. [CrossRef] [PubMed]
60. Yeo, S.Y.; Bratke, G.; Grüll, H. High Intensity Focused Ultrasound for Treatment of Bone Malignancies—20 Years of History. *Cancers* **2023**, *15*, 108. [CrossRef] [PubMed]
61. Lee, F.Y.; Latich, I.; Toombs, C.; Mungur, A.; Conway, D.; Alder, K.; Ibe, I.; Lindskog, D.; Friedlaender, G. Minimally Invasive Image-Guided Ablation, Osteoplasty, Reinforcement, and Internal Fixation (AORIF) for Osteolytic Lesions in the Pelvis and Periarticular Regions of Weight-Bearing Bones. *J. Vasc. Interv. Radiol.* **2020**, *31*, 649–658.e1. [CrossRef] [PubMed]
62. Jiang, W.; Friedlaender, G.; Lindskog, D.; Latich, I.; Lee, F.Y. Comparison of Percutaneous Interventional Ablation-Osteoplasty-Reinforcement-Internal Fixation (AORIF), Long Intramedullary Nailing, and Hemiarthroplasty for the Treatment of Focal Metastatic Osteolytic Lesions in the Femoral Head and Neck. *Cardiovasc. Interv. Radiol.* **2023**, *46*, 649–657. [CrossRef]
63. Morris, M.T.; Alder, K.D.; Moushey, A.; Munger, A.M.; Milligan, K.; Toombs, C.; Conway, D.; Lee, I.; Chen, F.; Tommasini, S.M.; et al. Biomechanical restoration of metastatic cancer-induced peri-acetabular bone defects by ablation-osteoplasty-reinforcement-internal fixation technique (AORIF): To screw or not to screw? *Clin. Biomech.* **2022**, *92*, 105565. [CrossRef]
64. Kim, H.J.; Zuckerman, S.L.; Cerpa, M.; Yeom, J.S.; Lehman, R.A.; Lenke, L.G. Incidence and Risk Factors for Complications and Mortality After Vertebroplasty or Kyphoplasty in the Osteoporotic Vertebral Compression Fracture—Analysis of 1,932 Cases from the American College of Surgeons National Surgical Quality Improvement. *Glob. Spine J.* **2022**, *12*, 1125–1134. [CrossRef] [PubMed]
65. Cavka, M.; Delimar, D.; Rezan, R.; Zigman, T.; Duric, K.S.; Cimic, M.; Dumic-Cule, I.; Prutki, M. Complications of Percutaneous Vertebroplasty: A Pictorial Review. *Medicina* **2023**, *59*, 1536. [CrossRef]

Journal of *Personalized Medicine*

MDPI

*Review*

# Genicular Artery Embolization: A New Tool for the Management of Refractory Osteoarthritis-Related Knee Pain

**Marco Femia [1,*], Carlo Valenti Pittino [1], Enrico Maria Fumarola [1], Marco Tramarin [1], Maurizio Papa [2], Francesco Giurazza [3], Antonio Pio Francioso [2], Davide Fior [4], Lorenzo Paolo Moramarco [4], Guido Antonini [5], Ruggero Vercelli [1] and Maurizio Cariati [1]**

1 Interventional Radiology Unit, ASST Santi Paolo Carlo, 20122 Milan, Italy
2 Complex Unit of Radiology, Department of Diagnostic, ASST Lodi, 26900 Lodi, Italy
3 Interventional Radiology Department, AORN "A. Cardarelli", 80100 Naples, Italy
4 Department of Radiology, Sant'Anna Hospital, ASST Lariana, 22100 Como, Italy
5 Department of Orthopedic and Traumatology, ASST Santi Paolo e Carlo, San Carlo Borromeo Hospital, 20122 Milan, Italy
* Correspondence: marco.femia@asst-santipaolocarlo.it

**Abstract:** Osteoarthritis (OA) of the knee is a prevalent cause of chronic pain and disability, particularly affecting women. While traditionally attributed to chronic wear and tear, recent evidence highlights multifactorial pathogenesis involving low-grade inflammation and neoangiogenesis. Current therapeutic options include physical therapy, pharmacotherapy, and total knee arthroplasty (TKA). However, a subset of patients remain symptomatic despite conservative measures, necessitating the development of minimally invasive interventions. Genicular artery embolization (GAE) emerges as a promising option, targeting neovascularization and inflammatory processes in OA. This paper reviews the pathophysiological basis, patient selection criteria, procedural details, and outcomes of GAE. Notably, GAE demonstrates efficacy in relieving knee pain and improving function in patients refractory to conventional therapy. While further research is warranted to elucidate its long-term outcomes and compare it with existing modalities, GAE represents a novel approach in the management of symptomatic knee OA, potentially delaying or obviating the need for surgical intervention. Here, we synthesize the relevant literature, technical details of the procedure, and future perspectives. Moreover, the success of GAE prompts the exploration of transarterial embolization in other musculoskeletal conditions, underscoring the evolving role of interventional radiology in personalized pain management strategies.

**Keywords:** genicular artery embolization; GAE; knee osteoarthritis; knee pain

## 1. Introduction

Osteoarthritis is a leading cause of adult chronic pain and disability, with the knee representing the most common site of osteoarthritis [1]. It has an age standardized prevalence of about 4300 cases per 100,000 individuals, with women being more affected than men [2].

Although chronic "wear and tear" is traditionally thought to be the main mechanism, new evidence suggests that the pathogenesis of knee osteoarthritis is multifactorial, with low-grade inflammation and neoangiogenesis playing a key role [3]. The treatment armamentarium for the management of symptomatic knee osteoarthritis (KO) includes physical therapy, drugs, such as non-steroidal anti-inflammatory drugs (NSAIDs), intra-articular infiltrations of hyaluronic acid and corticosteroids, and, eventually, total knee arthroplasty (TKA). A broad group of patients remain symptomatic despite therapeutic efforts, with a subset showing mild to moderate articular degeneration which would not warrant surgical joint replacement [4]. Thus, there is a need to develop new, effective, minimally invasive treatments to address symptomatic mild to moderate KO resistant to conservative therapies.

## 2. Pathophysiology

### 2.1. Inflammation

Inflammation can be either acute or chronic, when long-lasting, in response to injury.

While acute inflammation is locally characterized by fluid effusion with granulocytic cells, accompanied by systemic responses such as fever, leukocytosis, protein catabolism, and serum C-reactive protein elevation, chronic inflammation is usually more subtle and characterized by tissue monocytic infiltration [5–7].

Acute inflammation may resolve or evolve into chronic inflammation while the latter can also start directly from the very beginning [6,8].

### 2.2. Angiogenesis

The synovial joint has a structure which allows both stability and movement. The normal synovial lining is highly vascular, feeding the avascular articular cartilage [9].

Angiogenesis is the development of new capillaries from pre-existing blood vessels. Inflammatory cells produce proangiogenic factors which stimulate the growth and invasion of new blood vessels, which ease inflammatory cell infiltration. In osteoarthritis, angiogenesis seems to maintain rather than trigger inflammation [7].

Angiogenesis results from a cascade of processes and is involved in different pathologic processes such as chronic inflammation and the metastatic spread of tumors.

Angiogenic factors, such as vascular endothelial growth factor (VEGF), angiopoietin-1 (Ang-1), nerve growth factor (NGF), and basic fibroblast growth factor (bFGF), released within the synovium by many inflammatory cells, stimulate local endothelial cells in secreting proteolytic enzymes, which degrade the endothelial basement membrane and the perivascular extracellular matrix. This allows endothelial cells to proliferate and migrate to develop a primary sprout which, in turn, leads to the development of capillary loops. The subsequent synthesis of a basement membrane around the vascular loops ultimately leads to capillary formation [10].

The microenvironment of inflammatory areas of the synovial membrane seems to have higher levels of pro-inflammatory cytokines than normal areas. In fact, researchers demonstrated a higher secretion of pro-inflammatory mediators, such as VEGF, interleukin-6 (IL-6), interleukin-8 (IL-8), by synovial fibroblast cells of inflammatory areas and a lower secretion of trombospondin-1, which is an anti-angiogenic factor [11].

Pro-inflammatory cytokines such as IL-6, IL-8, and tumor necrosis factor-a (TNF-a) are involved in OA as well as in neovascularization, either directly stimulating the process or promoting the secretion of VEGF [12]. In regard to neovascularization, VEGF seems to play a key role in the angiogenic process, promoting both the proliferation and migration of endothelial cells [13].

The final effect of these mediators is an increased vascularity in the synovium seen in OA patients and an invasion of cartilage by new vessels from the underlying bone [14]. As a result, patients with OA of all grades experience a thickening of the synovial lining cell layer, neovascularization, and inflammatory cell infiltration of the synovial membranes, changes that are more evident in severe OA [14,15]. The awareness of the importance of the angiogenetic process stimulated the need to develop new lines of research which addressed the treatment of neovessels in the osteoarthritic joints, leading to the development of the genicular artery embolization (GAE) procedure.

## 3. Indications and Patient Preparation

The therapeutic efforts of painful knee osteoarthritis traditionally focused on physical therapy (such as muscle strengthening, exercises, and stretching), anti-inflammatory drugs (such as NSAIDs, corticosteroids, and opioids) and intra-articular infiltrations of hyaluronic acid and corticosteroids. However, the last traditional option for patients not responding to these therapies is TKA [4]. The non-invasive nature of physical therapy justifies its role as the first line therapy for the disease. When ineffective, patients start medications and interventions. NSAIDs often provide minimal pain relief and their chronic overuse raises the risk of kidney and hepatic failure; moreover, opioids may induce addiction and corticosteroids give a high risk of both metabolic impairment and osteoporosis. Intra-articular injections of hyaluronic acid and corticosteroids, although minimally invasive, often provide limited efficacy over the long term, thus requiring repetitive sessions [4,16]. Due to the longer life expectancy of patients, the objective of the genicular artery embolization procedure is to postpone surgical replacement as much as possible, or to offer another therapeutic chance to those patients not willing to undergo or not eligible for TKA.

The main case series include young or older adults with moderate to severe knee pain (i.e., a visual analogue scale (VAS, from 0 to 10) higher than 4) who did not experience benefit from at least 3 months of continuous conservative therapies [17–20]. Moreover, the assessment of the Western Ontario and McMaster Universities Osteoarthritis Index (WOMAC) preoperatively is suggested to understand the baseline symptoms and compare the result with those obtained after the treatment to understand its effectiveness [21,22].

To be proposed for GAE, patients need to undergo plain radiography in order to assess their Kellgren–Lawrence (KL) grade. KL grading is a five-grade system, published in 1957, based on plain radiography, which evaluates the severity of articular osteoarthrosis changes [23]. Usually, eligible patients include KL grade 1 to 3, while KL grade 4 patients are proposed for TKA unless they refuse or they are considered inoperable; in such cases, GAE may be proposed to improve symptoms although the literature on high-grade osteoarthritis is still insufficient. Pre-operative magnetic resonance imaging (MRI) without contrast medium (Figure 1) is suggested to exclude other sources of knee pain [20,24]; however, some authors suggest to complete the MRI study with post-contrast T1-weighted sequences [19].

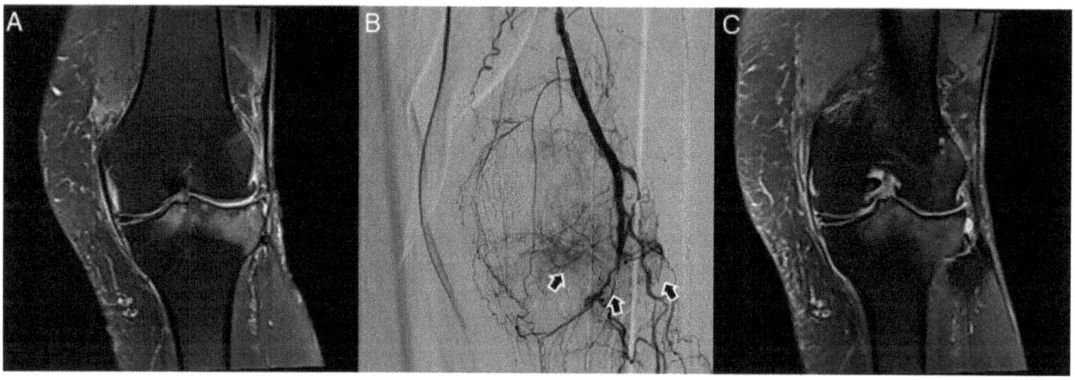


**Figure 1.** Magnetic resonance imaging and angiographic findings in an 87-year-old patient affected by osteoarthritis. The patient had undergone multiple conventional therapies over the years, including joint infiltrations and oral analgesics. She was not considered a candidate for TKA due to high surgical risk. Coronal fat-saturated T2-weighted MRI (**A**) shows diffuse oedema in the lateral compartment of the tibia. DSA performed at the femoral-popliteal transition (**B**) shows an area of hypervascularisation (blush) in the lateral compartment of the tibia (arrows) corresponding to the MRI finding. Magnetic resonance imaging conducted 4 months post embolization (**C**) exhibits a notable attenuation of bone marrow oedema; clinically, the patient reported diminished symptomatic pain and achieved unaided ambulation.

The additional value of post-contrast MRI images is to identify the areas of synovial hypervascularization, with the possibility to match them with clinical data and intraprocedural findings in order to guide the embolization procedure [25].

Peripheral arterial disease (PAD) represents one of the main contraindications because geniculate arteries play an important role as collateral circulation in case of popliteal and below-the-knee artery atherosclerotic occlusion, and patients with PAD may rely on these vessels to sustain leg perfusion [26]. In addition, severe PAD may complicate the procedure due to eventual genicular artery stenosis with a higher risk of arterial dissection, especially when treating those arteries branching off perpendicularly. Thus, a careful evaluation of peripheral pulses is mandatory while arterial duplex ultrasound is usually reserved to doubtful situations. It is also important to rule out general contraindications to arteriography by investigating baseline renal and coagulative function and possible allergy to iodinated contrast medium. Finally, due to the relatively high percentage of transient skin mottling occurrence, it is important to perform a pre-intervention dermatologic evaluation of the knee region.

## 4. Local Vascular Anatomy

The genicular arteries are a network of vessels that supply blood to the knee joint region.

These arteries include the descending genicular artery (DGA), superior lateral genicular artery (SLGA), superior medial genicular artery (SMGA), middle genicular artery (MGA), inferior lateral genicular artery (ILGA), inferior medial genicular artery (IMGA), recurrent anterior tibial artery (RATA), and superior patellar artery (SPA). The conventional genicular artery anatomy is illustrated in the figure below (Figure 2).

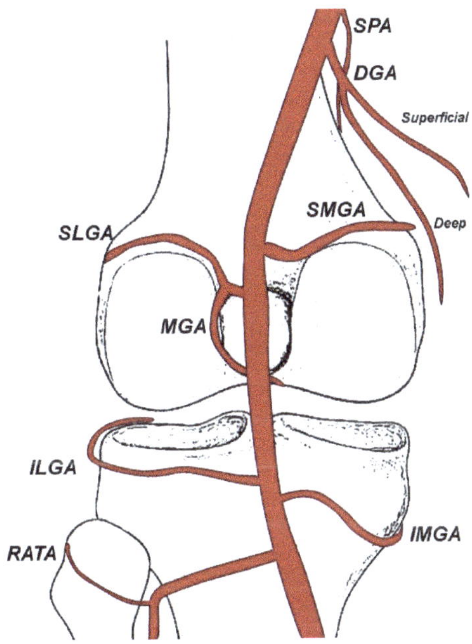


**Figure 2.** The typical branching patterns of the genicular arteries.

The medial portion of the knee receives its primary blood supply from the DGA, SMGA, and IMGA. The DGA originates from the superficial distal femoral artery, and bifurcates into a superficial (myocutaneous) branch, known as the superficial medial saphenous branch, and a deeper, more convoluted lateral musculoarticular branch, that perfuses the joint.

The SMGA divides into one branch supplying the vastus medialis, while the other branch supplies the femur and knee joint.

The IMGA supplies the upper end of the tibia and knee joint.

The MGA may originate from a common point with the LSGA or isolated. It provides perfusion to both the anterior and posterior cruciate ligaments and to the synovial membrane of the knee.

The SPA has a variable origin from the DGA or directly from the femoral artery and has a characteristic serpiginous course to the anterior part of the knee, toward the patellofemoral compartment.

The lateral compartment of the knee is mainly perfused by the SLGA, ILGA, and RATA. The SLGA is divided into a superficial branch that supplies the vastus lateralis and a deep branch that supplies the lower part of the femur and knee joint.

The ILGA ends with branches that anastomose with the IMGA, SLGA, and RATA [22].

The medial joint compartment is the weight-bearing portion of the joint and therefore the one most frequently affected by degenerative osteoarthritis [27]. Consequently, the arterial branches of this compartment are most often targeted for embolization.

Significant variation in genicular artery anatomy exists and holds crucial significance for interventional radiologists. A recent cadaveric study [28] provided a comprehensive classification system for variations in branching patterns and the presence of arterial anastomoses. This thorough understanding of anatomy is paramount for ensuring the safety and efficacy of interventions.

The presence of arterial anastomoses is particularly noteworthy during embolization procedures due to the potential risk of non-target embolization via these connections. In their study, O'Grady et al. [28] observed that the SMGA shared an origin with the MGA in 25% of cases. Non-target embolization (NTE) to the MGA may result in damage to the cruciate ligaments. In addition, anastomosis between the DGA and SMGA was found in 85% of cases, with a mean diameter of 850 microns, representing another risk of NTE.

Intraoperative cone-beam computer tomography (CBCT) stands as a crucial supplement to conventional angiography and CT angiography, providing a more comprehensive understanding of genicular artery anatomy. In comparison to digital subtraction angiography (DSA), CBCT has superior resolution capabilities, which allow it to accurately identify complex structures such as small-caliber vessels and anastomoses [29]. The high anatomic definition offered by CBCT plays a key role in interventional planning and in ensuring the accuracy and safety of procedures targeting the genicular arteries.

In their study, E. Callese et al. [29] identified through CBCT four genicular artery branching variants: Type 1: common trunk of SLGA and MGA; Type 2: independent origins; Type 3: common trunk of the SLGA, MGA, and SMGA; and Type 4: common trunk of the MGA and SMGA.

Understanding the anatomy and variants of the geniculate arteries is essential for interventional radiologists performing procedures such as GAE, in terms of treatment efficacy and to minimize complications.

## 5. Embolization Procedure

GAE is an elective symptom-related procedure which implies the treatment of painful regions showing "tumor blush" appearance at selective and/or superselective angiography. As such, it is important to ask the patient to point to the most painful sites in order to place radiopaque markers on the skin, useful to guide the embolization.

Before the procedure, intravenous antibiotic prophylaxis should be administered (commonly, 2 g of cephazolin). The angiographic suite should be prepared for peripheral angiography, so it could be useful to reverse head-to-feet the usual patient position.

Ultrasound-guided vascular access is recommended and it may be performed either antegrade or contralateral retrograde, in case of a prominent belly or atherosclerotic plaques on the common femoral artery.

The introducer sheath can be selected on the basis of the operator preference. The most common introducer sheaths used are standard 4 French sheath and the 3 French sheath, commonly included in the micropuncture set. In the latter case, the operator renounces the use of an intermediate 4 French diagnostic catheter.

Then, a digital subtraction angiography (DSA) of the superficial femoral artery at the knee level is performed by injecting either through the sheath or through the diagnostic catheter 15 mL of iodinated contrast agent at a flow rate of 3 to 4 mL/s. It is important to make a long-lasting angiographic run to observe the parenchymal phase. "Tumor blush" may not be visible through the femoral or popliteal injection, so a superselective angiography of the arteries supplying the painful region is necessary. Superselective catheterization should be performed with a 2.4 Fr or thinner microcatheter in order to facilitate a distal embolization avoiding spasm.

It is important to identify dangerous anastomoses such as those with popliteal artery, or other collaterals which can lead to off-target embolization, such as cutaneous collaterals. In this setting, the use of cone-beam computed tomography (CBCT) is helpful due to its three-dimensional view and its higher resolution compared to the two-dimensional images of DSA.

Before starting the embolization, an ice pack should be placed on the skin of the target region. This significantly reduces the risk of skin ulceration by inducing the vasoconstriction of skin collaterals [20]. Once the microcatheter is advanced within the target vessel, a DSA is necessary to demonstrate the "tumor-like blush" appearance, and the embolic material is slowly injected until pruning of the neovascularity is obtained and pathologic hyperemia is no longer seen, while preserving the patency of the parent vessel (Figure 3).

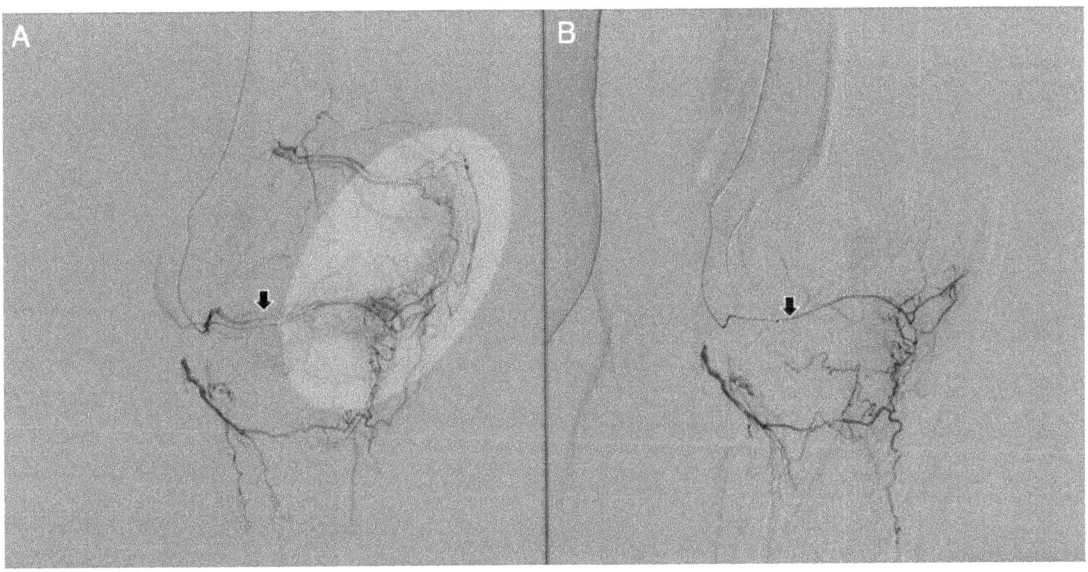


**Figure 3.** Selective angiography of the ILGA using a microcatheter (arrow). Initial angiographic image (**A**) shows hypervascular "blush" (highlighted in blue oval). After the delivery of 100–300 micron microspheres, the angiogram (**B**) shows "pruning" of the artery with patent parent vessel. The patient had no procedural adverse events.

As the amount of embolic material is usually small, it is suggested to inject 0.2 increments of embolic material, followed by saline. In addition, between each bolus, DSA is necessary to recognize the appropriate embolization point. Every vessel supplying the painful region should be studied and treated if "tumor-like blush" is recognized. Finally, the hemostasis of the vascular access can be achieved either through an occlusion device or manual compression.

*Embolic Materials*

The first case series about the treatment of refractory knee pain secondary to osteoarthritis, published by Okuno et al., described the use of both temporary and permanent embolic agents.

Okuno and colleagues employed imipenem/cilastatin sodium as a temporary embolic and permanent 75 mm microparticles.

Imipenem/cilastatin is an antibiotic which demonstrates slight solubility in water, and, when suspended in contrast agent, constitutes 10 to 70 mm particles that have an embolic effect [17].

The results of Okuno et al. showed the good efficacy of both embolic materials without major adverse events [17].

Unfortunately, imipenem/cilastatin sodium is not readily available everywhere with this indication. As such, many authors focused on the use of microparticles with good results but obtaining a permanent embolization [17–20].

However, the possibility to use a temporary embolic agent seemed a great opportunity in order to reduce the risk of ischemic adverse events. In a recent trial by Sapoval and colleagues, the authors decided to study the efficacy of an ethiodized oil-based emulsion between the temporary embolic agent Lipiodol Ultra-Fluid (Guerbet) and the contrast agent ioversol 300 mgI/mL in a 1:3 mixture which was found in a previous reserved study, by their group, to be able to embolize vessels for about 10 min. In their LipioJoint-1 trial, they obtained good clinical results and no embolic material-specific adverse events. At the same time, Min et al. tested another temporary embolic material based on the gelatin sponge widely used for the temporary embolization of bleeding vessels or at the end of hepatic chemoembolization to obtain stasis within the treated vessels, which is said to be degraded within 24–48 h into the bloodstream [30]. A recent metanalysis compared the performance of temporary and permanent embolic agents. The results did not show significant differences in patients' outcomes between the two groups [31]. However, to date, the experience is still limited and there is no wide consensus yet on which embolic material is safer and more efficacious, although results on both matters seem to be comparable.

## 6. Expected Outcome and Complications

### 6.1. Expected Outcome

The results of GAE for the treatment of refractory knee pain secondary to osteoarthritis are usually evaluated with the use of validated self-administered scales either general, such as VAS, or specific for hip and knee osteoarthritis as in the case of WOMAC. While the former exclusively evaluates pain, WOMAC also takes into consideration articular functionality and stiffness. Some authors decided to use the Knee Injury and Osteoarthritis Outcome Score (KOOS), which is a more recent questionnaire evaluating symptoms related to osteoarthritis and their impact on patients' quality of life [32–34].

In the main case series published so far, both VAS and WOMAC scores were substantially reduced within the first month [17–20,35–37], often remaining low until the third month (Figures 4 and 5).

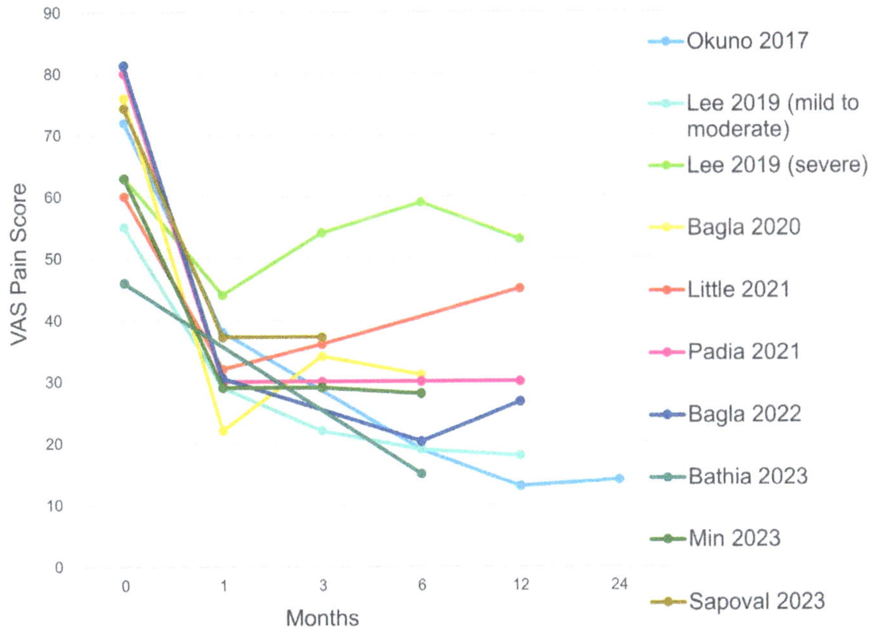


**Figure 4.** VAS score during the follow-up period of the main case series [18–20,30,35–38].

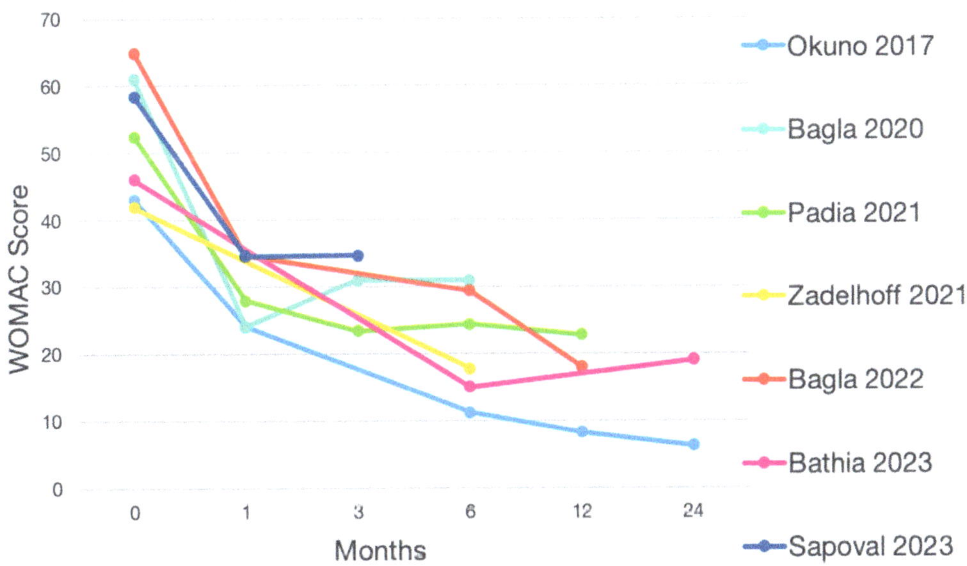


**Figure 5.** WOMAC score during the follow-up period of the main case series [19,20,36–40].

However, in some papers, a small rebound in pain and articular symptoms was registered after the first month [18,19,35]. This finding can be due to the patient's characteristics.

In the paper by Lee et al. only the subset affected by severe osteoarthritis experienced symptom rebound, while the subset of patients with mild to moderate KO had a long lasting benefit which remained up to 12 months, suggesting a poorer outcome in more advanced KO [35]. Choi and colleagues observed a significant difference in response among KL grades, identifying a grading ≥3 as a predictor of poor response [24], and thus highlighting the importance of OA severity. Nevertheless, these results are in contrast with the subsequent experience by Padia and colleagues, whose study population included up to 40% of KL grade 4 patients. In their study, 60% and 53% of patients registered a decrease of at least 50% in VAS and WOMAC scores, respectively, at 1 month, and the percentage rose up to 68% in both categories at the 1-year follow-up [20]. The main difference between these experiences is that while the group of Padia obtained vessel embolization through non-resorbable particles, Lee et al. and Choi and colleagues employed IM/CS and a combination of IM/CS and gelatin sponge, which are all temporary embolic agent. Finally, the most recent case series published by Sapoval and colleagues employed another type of resorbable embolic agent based on the ethiodized oil Lipiodol Ultra-Fluid (Guerbet, Paris, France) [39]. They exclusively enrolled KL 3 and 4 patients, obtaining a mean reduction in VAS of 50% for the three-month follow-up. Although promising, this result needs to be confirmed over the long term.

In conclusion, based on the most recent studies, patients affected by OA-related knee pain can expect a 30% to 50% reduction in VAS and WOMAC scores, which in most cases lasts up to 6 months, and can protract up to 1 or 2 years. The effectiveness of GAE is less predictable in more severe settings, particularly in KL 4 grades, for which research results are still poor and controversial.

### *6.2. Complications*

Most of the adverse events in GAE are secondary to non-target embolization. Indeed, those most observed across the main case series published so far are skin mottling and discoloration, which can occur in up to 65% of cases [19,30], and this is thought to be due to the embolization of small perforators supplying the skin, which cannot be avoided. Due to the undesired embolization of cutaneous branches, Padia et al. [20] reported seven cases of focal skin ulceration (<1 cm), which resolved spontaneously without sequelae. Since the group decided to adjust the embolization protocol by applicating an ice pack over the target area before the procedure, no more events of skin necrosis occurred. At the 3-month MRI, the same group observed 2 cases out of 40 enrolled patients of clinically asymptomatic focal bone infarct smaller than 2 cm.

Two studies reported three cases of numbness in the below-the-knee area, which resolved in two weeks after the administration of gabapentin [19,36]. Although the embolization is usually minimal, Lee et al. registered one case of mild fever which spontaneously subsided in 1 day [35].

Finally, arterial access can be a source of complications as in other endovascular interventions. Although some cases of puncture site hematomas are exclusively reported in the literature [17,19,20,30,34,35], it is always necessary to pay attention to antegrade arterial punctures, which can give origin to arterial dissection and occlusion.

## 7. Transarterial Embolization in Other Musculoskeletal Conditions

The application of GAE also demonstrated successful results in the setting of recurrent hemarthrosis after TKA. This is an uncommon condition (0.3–1.6%); however, it is usually refractory to conservative treatment, and surgical revision is often required to obtain a definitive resolution [41,42]. GAE offers a minimally invasive solution with high rates of clinical success ranging from 76% to 89%, occasionally requiring more than one procedure [43].

Beyond knee-related conditions, a wide variety of musculoskeletal disorders can lead to chronic musculoskeletal pain, such as low back pain, hip pain, and rheumatoid and osteoarthritis (OA)-associated joint pain. The main symptom in patients with chronic musculoskeletal disorders is intense pain, which is often accompanied by stiffness. This frequently leads to sleep alterations, fatigue, reduced activity, mood impairment, and severe disability, with a significant impact on the quality of life.

Transarterial embolization (TAE) has been employed over time to treat many other pathologic musculoskeletal conditions, although data on its application in different joints and tendons are still very limited [44]. Firstly, TAE for musculoskeletal pain was employed by Okuno and colleagues to treat tendinopathy and enthesopathy refractory to nonsurgical management [45], even earlier than its application for the treatment of knee OA. They studied TAE in seven patients with tendinopathy and enthesopathy located at different sites (one patellar tendinopathy, two rotator cuff tendinopathies, one plantar fasciitis, one lateral epicondylitis, one iliotibial band syndrome, and one Achilles insertion tendinopathy), all united by recalcitrant pain. They registered a reduction in VAS scores greater than 85% for the entire follow-up period (4 months). The impressive success of this experience encouraged other groups to evaluate this technique in other musculoskeletal painful conditions. One of the most successful sites was the hip joint, with a great clinical success reported in a case report by Correa and colleagues [46], who registered complete pain resolution the day after the procedure, which was maintained up to the 4-month follow-up visit. Two years later, the same group published a more extensive experience on the treatment of painful hip joint, confirming the efficacy of TAE in the control of hip pain related to osteoarthritis and greater trochanteric pain syndrome [47]. Finally, TAE was also successfully employed in trapeziometacarpal and finger osteoarthritis, shoulder osteoarthritis, adhesive capsulitis, and many other conditions.

## 8. Future Directions and Conclusions

Genicular artery embolization (GAE) stands at the forefront of a new era in knee pain management, offering a personalized therapeutic approach through collaboration between interventional radiologists and orthopedic surgeons. In the treatment of refractory knee pain secondary to osteoarthritis (OA), GAE presents a promising alternative for patients who have exhausted conventional minimally invasive options, avoiding the necessity for suboptimal surgical interventions or enduring chronic pain.

The efficacy of GAE in alleviating knee pain is underscored by its impact on validated self-administered scales, such as the Visual Analog Scale (VAS) and the Western Ontario and McMaster Universities Osteoarthritis Index (WOMAC). Studies have shown significant reductions in pain and improvement in joint functionality, often sustained for months following the procedure. However, variability in outcomes exists, particularly in more severe cases of OA, emphasizing the need for further research to identify optimal candidates and standardize technical protocols.

Future investigations should focus on elucidating the long-term durability of pain relief, functional improvement, and potential adverse events associated with GAE. Additionally, understanding the procedure's impact on joint health and its role in the progression of osteoarthritis is paramount. Establishing comprehensive pre-operative evaluation criteria and follow-up protocols will not only optimize patient outcomes but also minimize unnecessary costs.

A holistic comparison between GAE, traditional pharmacotherapy, intra-articular injections, and surgery could provide invaluable insights into the most appropriate treatment modality for knee osteoarthritis. Furthermore, exploring GAE's potential to interrupt the vicious cycle of neoangiogenesis and inflammation may hold the key to slowing disease progression.

Finally, the success of GAE should encourage researchers to study the role of TAE in the management of other painful musculoskeletal conditions in order to legitimize its application as a frontline therapy of chronic musculoskeletal pain.

In conclusion, GAE heralds a paradigm shift in knee pain management, offering patients a ray of hope for improved quality of life through less invasive and more targeted interventions. As research advances and clinical experience grows, GAE has the potential to revolutionize the therapeutic landscape, providing a tailored approach to each patient's unique needs and circumstances.

**Author Contributions:** Conceptualization, M.F.; writing—original draft preparation, M.F., C.V.P., E.M.F., M.T., M.P. and F.G.; writing—review and editing, C.V.P., E.M.F., M.T., L.P.M. and R.V.; visualization, A.P.F., D.F. and G.A.; supervision, G.A., R.V. and M.C. All authors have read and agreed to the published version of the manuscript.

**Funding:** This research received no external funding.

**Institutional Review Board Statement:** Not applicable.

**Informed Consent Statement:** Not applicable.

**Data Availability Statement:** Not applicable.

**Conflicts of Interest:** The authors declare no conflicts of interest.

## References

1. Vina, E.R.; Kwoh, C.K. Epidemiology of Osteoarthritis: Literature Update. *Curr. Opin. Rheumatol.* **2018**, *30*, 160–167. [CrossRef]
2. Steinmetz, J.D.; Culbreth, G.T.; Haile, L.M.; Rafferty, Q.; Lo, J.; Fukutaki, K.G.; Cruz, J.A.; Smith, A.E.; Vollset, S.E.; Brooks, P.M.; et al. Global, Regional, and National Burden of Osteoarthritis, 1990–2020 and Projections to 2050: A Systematic Analysis for the Global Burden of Disease Study 2021. *Lancet Rheumatol.* **2023**, *5*, e508–e522. [CrossRef] [PubMed]
3. Tyagi, R.; Ahmed, S.S.; Koethe, Y.; Raskind, A.; Ahmed, O. Genicular Artery Embolization for Primary Knee Osteoarthritis. *Semin. Interv. Radiol.* **2022**, *39*, 125–129. [CrossRef] [PubMed]
4. Bannuru, R.R.; Osani, M.C.; Vaysbrot, E.E.; Arden, N.K.; Bennell, K.; Bierma-Zeinstra, S.M.A.; Kraus, V.B.; Lohmander, L.S.; Abbott, J.H.; Bhandari, M.; et al. OARSI Guidelines for the Non-Surgical Management of Knee, Hip, and Polyarticular Osteoarthritis. *Osteoarthr. Cartil.* **2019**, *27*, 1578–1589. [CrossRef] [PubMed]
5. Bijlsma, J.W.J.; Berenbaum, F.; Lafeber, F.P.J.G. Osteoarthritis: An Update with Relevance for Clinical Practice. *Lancet* **2011**, *377*, 2115–2126. [CrossRef] [PubMed]
6. Poudel, P.; Goyal, A.; Lappin, S.L. Inflammatory Arthritis. In *StatPearls [Internet]*; StatPearls Publishing: Tampa/St. Petersburg, FL, USA, 2023.
7. Bonnet, C.S.; Walsh, D.A. Osteoarthritis, Angiogenesis and Inflammation. *Rheumatology* **2005**, *44*, 7–16. [CrossRef] [PubMed]
8. He, Y.; Li, Z.; Alexander, P.G.; Ocasio-Nieves, B.D.; Yocum, L.; Lin, H.; Tuan, R.S. Pathogenesis of Osteoarthritis: Risk Factors, Regulatory Pathways in Chondrocytes, and Experimental Models. *Biology* **2020**, *9*, 194. [CrossRef] [PubMed]
9. Haywood, L.; Walsh, D.A. Vasculature of the Normal and Arthritic Synovial Joint. *Histol. Histopathol.* **2001**, *16*, 277–284. [CrossRef] [PubMed]
10. Henrotin, Y.; Pesesse, L.; Lambert, C. Targeting the Synovial Angiogenesis as a Novel Treatment Approach to Osteoarthritis. *Ther. Adv. Musculoskelet. Dis.* **2014**, *6*, 20–34. [CrossRef] [PubMed]
11. Lambert, C.; Mathy-Hartert, M.; Dubuc, J.-E.; Montell, E.; Vergés, J.; Munaut, C.; Noël, A.; Henrotin, Y. Characterization of Synovial Angiogenesis in Osteoarthritis Patients and Its Modulation by Chondroitin Sulfate. *Arthritis Res. Ther.* **2012**, *14*, R58. [CrossRef]
12. de Lange-Brokaar, B.J.E.; Ioan-Facsinay, A.; van Osch, G.J.V.M.; Zuurmond, A.-M.; Schoones, J.; Toes, R.E.M.; Huizinga, T.W.J.; Kloppenburg, M. Synovial Inflammation, Immune Cells and Their Cytokines in Osteoarthritis: A Review. *Osteoarthr. Cartil.* **2012**, *20*, 1484–1499. [CrossRef] [PubMed]
13. Notch Signalling Pathways Mediate Synovial Angiogenesis in Response to Vascular Endothelial Growth Factor and Angiopoietin 2—PubMed. Available online: https://pubmed.ncbi.nlm.nih.gov/23161900/ (accessed on 21 February 2024).
14. Stephens, R.W.; Ghosh, P.; Taylor, T.K. The Pathogenesis of Osteoarthrosis. *Med. Hypotheses* **1979**, *5*, 809–816. [CrossRef] [PubMed]
15. Sellam, J.; Berenbaum, F. The Role of Synovitis in Pathophysiology and Clinical Symptoms of Osteoarthritis. *Nat. Rev. Rheumatol.* **2010**, *6*, 625–635. [CrossRef] [PubMed]
16. Roque, V.; Agre, M.; Barroso, J.; Brito, I. Managing Knee Ostheoarthritis: Efficacy of Hyaluronic Acid Injections. *Acta Reumatol. Port.* **2013**, *38*, 154–161. [PubMed]
17. Okuno, Y.; Korchi, A.M.; Shinjo, T.; Kato, S. Transcatheter Arterial Embolization as a Treatment for Medial Knee Pain in Patients with Mild to Moderate Osteoarthritis. *Cardiovasc. Intervent. Radiol.* **2015**, *38*, 336–343. [CrossRef] [PubMed]
18. Little, M.W.; Gibson, M.; Briggs, J.; Speirs, A.; Yoong, P.; Ariyanayagam, T.; Davies, N.; Tayton, E.; Tavares, S.; MacGill, S.; et al. Correction to: Genicular artEry embolizatioN in patiEnts with oSteoarthrItiS of the Knee (GENESIS) Using Permanent Microspheres: Interim Analysis. *Cardiovasc. Intervent. Radiol.* **2021**, *44*, 1153. [CrossRef] [PubMed]
19. Bagla, S.; Piechowiak, R.; Hartman, T.; Orlando, J.; Del Gaizo, D.; Isaacson, A. Genicular Artery Embolization for the Treatment of Knee Pain Secondary to Osteoarthritis. *J. Vasc. Interv. Radiol.* **2020**, *31*, 1096–1102. [CrossRef] [PubMed]
20. Padia, S.A.; Genshaft, S.; Blumstein, G.; Plotnik, A.; Kim, G.H.J.; Gilbert, S.J.; Lauko, K.; Stavrakis, A.I. Genicular Artery Embolization for the Treatment of Symptomatic Knee Osteoarthritis. *JBJS Open Access* **2021**, *6*, 85. [CrossRef]

21. McConnell, S.; Kolopack, P.; Davis, A.M. The Western Ontario and McMaster Universities Osteoarthritis Index (WOMAC): A Review of Its Utility and Measurement Properties. *Arthritis Rheum.* **2001**, *45*, 453–461. [CrossRef]
22. Poursalehian, M.; Bhia, I.; Ayati Firoozabadi, M.; Mortazavi, S.M.J. Genicular Artery Embolization for Knee Osteoarthritis: A Comprehensive Review. *JBJS Rev.* **2023**, *11*, 82. [CrossRef]
23. Kellgren, J.H.; Lawrence, J.S. Radiological Assessment of Osteo-Arthrosis. *Ann. Rheum. Dis.* **1957**, *16*, 494–502. [CrossRef] [PubMed]
24. Choi, J.W.; Ro, D.H.; Chae, H.D.; Kim, D.H.; Lee, M.; Hur, S.; Kim, H.-C.; Jae, H.J.; Chung, J.W. The Value of Preprocedural MR Imaging in Genicular Artery Embolization for Patients with Osteoarthritic Knee Pain. *J. Vasc. Interv. Radiol.* **2020**, *31*, 2043–2050. [CrossRef] [PubMed]
25. Korchi, A.M.; Cengarle-Samak, A.; Okuno, Y.; Martel-Pelletier, J.; Pelletier, J.P.; Boesen, M.; Doyon, J.; Bodson-Clermont, P.; Lussier, B.; Héon, H.; et al. Inflammation and Hypervascularization in a Large Animal Model of Knee Osteoarthritis: Imaging with Pathohistologic Correlation. *J. Vasc. Interv. Radiol.* **2019**, *30*, 1116–1127. [CrossRef]
26. Dua, A.; Desai, S.S.; Johnston, S.; Chinapuvvula, N.R.; Wade, C.E.; Fox, C.J.; Holcomb, J.B.; Coogan, S. The Impact of Geniculate Artery Collateral Circulation on Lower Limb Salvage Rates in Injured Patients. *Ann. Vasc. Surg.* **2016**, *30*, 258–262. [CrossRef] [PubMed]
27. Jones, R.K.; Chapman, G.J.; Findlow, A.H.; Forsythe, L.; Parkes, M.J.; Sultan, J.; Felson, D.T. A New Approach to Prevention of Knee Osteoarthritis: Reducing Medial Load in the Contralateral Knee. *J. Rheumatol.* **2013**, *40*, 309–315. [CrossRef] [PubMed]
28. O'Grady, A.; Welsh, L.; Gibson, M.; Briggs, J.; Speirs, A.; Little, M. Cadaveric and Angiographic Anatomical Considerations in the Genicular Arterial System: Implications for Genicular Artery Embolisation in Patients with Knee Osteoarthritis. *Cardiovasc. Intervent. Radiol.* **2022**, *45*, 80–90. [CrossRef] [PubMed]
29. Callese, T.E.; Cusumano, L.; Redwood, K.D.; Genshaft, S.; Plotnik, A.; Stewart, J.; Padia, S.A. Classification of Genicular Artery Anatomic Variants Using Intraoperative Cone-Beam Computed Tomography. *Cardiovasc. Intervent. Radiol.* **2023**, *46*, 628–634. [CrossRef] [PubMed]
30. Min, J.; Park, S.W.; Hwang, J.H.; Lee, J.K.; Lee, D.W.; Kwon, Y.W.; Shin, K.C. Evaluating the Safety and Effectiveness of Quick-Soluble Gelatin Sponge Particles for Genicular Artery Embolization for Chronic Knee Pain Associated with Osteoarthritis. *J. Vasc. Interv. Radiol.* **2023**, *34*, 1868–1874. [CrossRef]
31. Epelboym, Y.; Mandell, J.C.; Collins, J.E.; Burch, E.; Shiang, T.; Killoran, T.; Macfarlane, L.; Guermazi, A. Genicular Artery Embolization as a Treatment for Osteoarthritis Related Knee Pain: A Systematic Review and Meta-Analysis. *Cardiovasc. Intervent. Radiol.* **2023**, *46*, 760–769. [CrossRef]
32. Roos, E.M.; Roos, H.P.; Lohmander, L.S.; Ekdahl, C.; Beynnon, B.D. Knee Injury and Osteoarthritis Outcome Score (KOOS)—Development of a Self-Administered Outcome Measure. *J. Orthop. Sports Phys. Ther.* **1998**, *28*, 88–96. [CrossRef]
33. Collins, N.J.; Prinsen, C.A.C.; Christensen, R.; Bartels, E.M.; Terwee, C.B.; Roos, E.M. Knee Injury and Osteoarthritis Outcome Score (KOOS): Systematic Review and Meta-Analysis of Measurement Properties. *Osteoarthr. Cartil.* **2016**, *24*, 1317–1329. [CrossRef] [PubMed]
34. Landers, S.; Hely, R.; Hely, A.; Harrison, B.; Page, R.S.; Maister, N.; Gwini, S.M.; Gill, S.D. Genicular Artery Embolization for Early-Stage Knee Osteoarthritis: Results from a Triple-Blind Single-Centre Randomized Controlled Trial. *Bone Jt. Open* **2023**, *4*, 158–167. [CrossRef] [PubMed]
35. Lee, S.H.; Hwang, J.H.; Kim, D.H.; So, Y.H.; Park, J.; Cho, S.B.; Kim, J.-E.; Kim, Y.J.; Hur, S.; Jae, H.J. Clinical Outcomes of Transcatheter Arterial Embolisation for Chronic Knee Pain: Mild-to-Moderate Versus Severe Knee Osteoarthritis. *Cardiovasc. Intervent. Radiol.* **2019**, *42*, 1530–1536. [CrossRef] [PubMed]
36. Bhatia, S.; Jalaeian, H.; Kumar, J.; Acharya, V.; Shibuya, M.; Bhatia, A.; Okuno, Y. Two-Year Outcomes Comparing Embosphere® Microspheres versus Imipenem Cilastatin for Genicular Artery Embolization in Patients with Moderate to Severe Knee Osteoarthritis. *Knee* **2023**, *41*, 38–47. [CrossRef] [PubMed]
37. Bagla, S.; Piechowiak, R.; Sajan, A.; Orlando, J.; Hartman, T.; Isaacson, A. Multicenter Randomized Sham Controlled Study of Genicular Artery Embolization for Knee Pain Secondary to Osteoarthritis. *J. Vasc. Interv. Radiol.* **2022**, *33*, 2–10.e2. [CrossRef] [PubMed]
38. Okuno, Y.; Korchi, A.M.; Shinjo, T.; Kato, S.; Kaneko, T. Midterm Clinical Outcomes and MR Imaging Changes after Transcatheter Arterial Embolization as a Treatment for Mild to Moderate Radiographic Knee Osteoarthritis Resistant to Conservative Treatment. *J. Vasc. Interv. Radiol.* **2017**, *28*, 995–1002. [CrossRef] [PubMed]
39. Sapoval, M.; Querub, C.; Pereira, H.; Pellerin, O.; Boeken, T.; Di Gaeta, A.; Ahmar, M.A.; Lefevre-Colau, M.-M.; Nguyen, C.; Daste, C.; et al. Genicular Artery Embolization for Knee Osteoarthritis: Results of the LipioJoint-1 Trial. *Diagn. Interv. Imaging* **2024**, *105*, 144–150. [CrossRef] [PubMed]
40. Van Zadelhoff, T.A.; Okuno, Y.; Bos, P.K.; Bierma-Zeinstra, S.M.A.; Krestin, G.P.; Moelker, A.; Oei, E.H.G. Association between Baseline Osteoarthritic Features on MR Imaging and Clinical Outcome after Genicular Artery Embolization for Knee Osteoarthritis. *J. Vasc. Interv. Radiol.* **2021**, *32*, 497–503. [CrossRef] [PubMed]
41. Ohdera, T.; Tokunaga, M.; Hiroshima, S.; Yoshimoto, E.; Matsuda, S. Recurrent Hemarthrosis after Knee Joint Arthroplasty: Etiology and Treatment. *J. Arthroplast.* **2004**, *19*, 157–161. [CrossRef]
42. Worland, R.L.; Jessup, D.E. Recurrent Hemarthrosis after Total Knee Arthroplasty. *J. Arthroplast.* **1996**, *11*, 977–978. [CrossRef]

43. Heller, D.B.; Beggin, A.E.; Lam, A.H.; Kohi, M.P.; Heller, M.B. Geniculate Artery Embolization: Role in Knee Hemarthrosis and Osteoarthritis. *RadioGraphics* **2022**, *42*, 289–301. [CrossRef] [PubMed]
44. Wang, B.; Liang, K.-W.; Chen, C.-H.; Wang, C.-K. Transcatheter Arterial Embolization for Alleviating Chronic Musculoskeletal Pain and Improving Physical Function: A Narrative Review. *Diagnostics* **2022**, *13*, 134. [CrossRef] [PubMed]
45. Okuno, Y.; Matsumura, N.; Oguro, S. Transcatheter Arterial Embolization Using Imipenem/Cilastatin Sodium for Tendinopathy and Enthesopathy Refractory to Nonsurgical Management. *J. Vasc. Interv. Radiol.* **2013**, *24*, 787–792. [CrossRef] [PubMed]
46. Correa, M.P.; Puton, R.C.; Saleh, J.N.; Noel, R.S.; Da Silva, L.H.P.; De Castro, D.M.; De Mello Bajesrki, J.C. Short-Term Follow-up of Embolization of Hip Synovitis. *CVIR Endovasc.* **2020**, *3*, 35. [CrossRef]
47. Correa, M.P.; Motta-Leal-Filho, J.M.; Junior, E.B.; Mansano, R.M.; Deuschle, J.S.; Puton, R.C.; De Souza Saleh, J.N.; Noel, R.S.; Bajerski, J.C. 6-Month Follow-up of Lateral Femoral Circumflex Artery Embolization to Control Pain Related to Hip Osteoarthritis and Greater Trochanteric Pain Syndrome. *Cardiovasc. Intervent. Radiol.* **2022**, *45*, 1710–1715. [CrossRef]

Journal of Personalized Medicine

MDPI

*Review*

# Damage Control Interventional Radiology in Liver Trauma: A Comprehensive Review

**Fabio Corvino [1,2,*], Francesco Giurazza [2], Paolo Marra [3], Anna Maria Ierardi [4], Antonio Corvino [5], Antonio Basile [6], Massimo Galia [1], Agostino Inzerillo [1] and Raffaella Niola [2]**

1. Section of Radiology, Department of Biomedicine, Neuroscience and Advanced Diagnostics (BiND), University Hospital "Paolo Giaccone", 90127 Palermo, Italy; massimo.galia@unipa.it (M.G.); agostino.inzerillo@unipa.it (A.I.)
2. Interventional Radiology Department, AORN "A. Cardarelli", 80131 Naples, Italy; francesco.giurazza@aocardarelli.it (F.G.); raffaella.niola@aocardarelli.it (R.N.)
3. Department of Radiology, Papa Giovanni XXIII Hospital, 24127 Bergamo, Italy; pmarra@asst-pg23.it
4. Department of Diagnostic and Interventional Radiology, Foundation IRCCS Cà Granda—Ospedale Maggiore Policlinico, 20122 Milan, Italy; annamaria.ierardi@policlinico.mi.it
5. Medical, Movement and Wellbeing Sciences Department, University of Naples "Parthenope", 80133 Naples, Italy; antonio.corvino@uniparthenope.it
6. Radiology Unit 1, Department of Medical Surgical Sciences and Advanced Technologies "GF Ingrassia", University Hospital "Policlinico-San Marco", University of Catania, 95123 Catania, Italy; basile.antonello73@gmail.com

* Correspondence: fabio.corvino@unipa.it; Tel.: +39-081-747-3828

**Abstract:** The liver is the second most common solid organ injured in blunt and penetrating abdominal trauma. Non-operative management (NOM) has become the standard of care for liver injuries in stable patients, where transarterial embolization (TAE) represents the main treatment, increasing success rates and avoiding invasive surgical procedures. In hemodynamically (HD) unstable patients, operative management (OM) is the standard of care. To date, there are no consensus guidelines about the endovascular treatment of patients with HD instability or in ones that responded to initial infusion therapy. A review of the literature was performed for published papers addressing the outcome of using TAE as the primary treatment for HD unstable/transient responder trauma liver patients with hemorrhagic vascular lesions, both as a single treatment and in combination with surgical treatment, focusing additionally on the different definitions used in the literature of unstable and transient responder patients. Our review demonstrated a good outcome in HD unstable/transient responder liver trauma patients treated with TAE but there still remains much debate about the definition of unstable and transient responder patients.

**Keywords:** liver trauma; damage control interventional radiology; transarterial embolization; hemodynamic instability

## 1. Introduction

Trauma is a global phenomenon; about 5 million people die worldwide each year due to an injury. Injuries also account for 17% of the disease burden in young adults aged between 15 and 60 years [1].

Interventional radiology (IR) plays a pivotal role in the management of trauma patients suffering from both blunt and penetrating injuries. In the last three decades, the focus on damage control resuscitation and damage control surgery has spared countless patients the morbidity of surgery, identifying which patients will benefit the most from a minimally invasive treatment strategy [2].

Prompt hemorrhage control with angioembolization (AE), as part of the damage control strategy, has been integrated into trauma resuscitation guidelines, as stated by the latest version of the Resources for Optimal Care of the Injured Patient from the American College of Surgeons Committee on Trauma [3].

The new concept of "damage control interventional radiology" (DCIR) proposed the availability of IR within less than 30 min in an emergency setting, trying to provide trauma patients with the best treatment as soon as possible to achieve the best possible outcome. In this context, even if according to the World Society of Emergency Surgery (WSES), hemodynamic (HD) unstable patients are an exclusive prerogative of surgical management, IR could be crucial in the management of HD unstable patients, especially for those who represent the transient responder class who need to receive endovascular hemostasis and subsequent resuscitation [4].

An earlier endovascular approach could also be possible due to the technological advancement achieved with the implementation of the trauma hybrid resuscitation suites that allow for the treatment of patients as soon as possible, both endovascular treatment alone or in combination with surgical procedures such as damage control surgery [5].

After the spleen, the most common solid organ injured in blunt and penetrating abdominal trauma is the liver; given its location and its relationship with other abdominal structures, the mortality rate is quite high at about 10–15% [6].

Non-operative management (NOM) is the current standard of care in the management of trauma liver patients who are HD stable and it consists of a basic "wait and see" attitude combined with blood replacement and systemic support. Imaging advancement has a major role in the success rate of NOM because it allows us to identify the injury grade, the presence of arterial hemorrhage and/or concomitant venous injury, which are crucial in the management algorithm [7]. To date, WSES classification in liver trauma patients with arterial hemorrhage or early pseudoaneurysm suggest AE as the primary treatment only in HD stable patients [8].

HD unstable and non-responder patients should undergo operative management (OM). Moreover, there is a "gray area" between stable and unstable patients, known as "transient responder patients", in which NOM should be considered only in selected settings that provide the immediate availability of both surgeons and interventional radiologists, with continuous monitoring, ideally in an intensive care unit or emergency room setting [8].

The purpose of this systematic review is to determine the safety and efficacy of AE as the primary treatment for HD unstable or transient responder trauma liver patients with hemorrhagic vascular lesions, both as a single treatment and in combination with surgical treatment, focusing additionally on the different definitions of HD instability.

## 2. Materials and Methods

A literature review with a focus primarily on AE in the treatment of vascular lesions due to liver trauma, both blunt and penetrating trauma, in HD unstable patients was conducted from January 1980 to January 2024.

A systematic literature search was performed using PubMed, Google Scholar and the Cochrane Central Register of Controlled Trials databases for studies published on the role of IR in the management of liver trauma in HD unstable patients, both as a single treatment or in combination with surgical treatment. Medical subject headings (MeSH) and database-specific search terms for "liver trauma", "liver embolization", "hemodynamic status" and "damage control interventional radiology" were combined as follows: ((hepatic) OR (liver)) AND (trauma) AND (embolization) OR (embolisation) OR (angioembolization) AND (hemodynamic) AND (unstable); ((((((hepatic) OR (liver)) AND (trauma)) AND (embolization)) OR (embolisation)) OR (angioembolisation)) AND (hemodynamic)) AND (unstable); (((hepatic) OR (liver)) AND (trauma)) AND (damage control interventional radiology)

Supplemented articles were implemented by the ones obtained from the reference list of all relevant articles. We included only articles in the English language where it was possible to access to the full content.

Preferred Reporting Items for Systematic Reviews (PRISMA) (Figure 1) was used as the reference for data collection and the search was performed between December 2023 and January 2024, including all of the articles published until January 2024. Our review included all of the studies that evaluated the efficacy, safety and feasibility of endovascular treatment in HD unstable patients with liver trauma hemorrhage, focusing especially on the hemodynamic parameters from a more clinical perspective of the interventional radiology treatment.

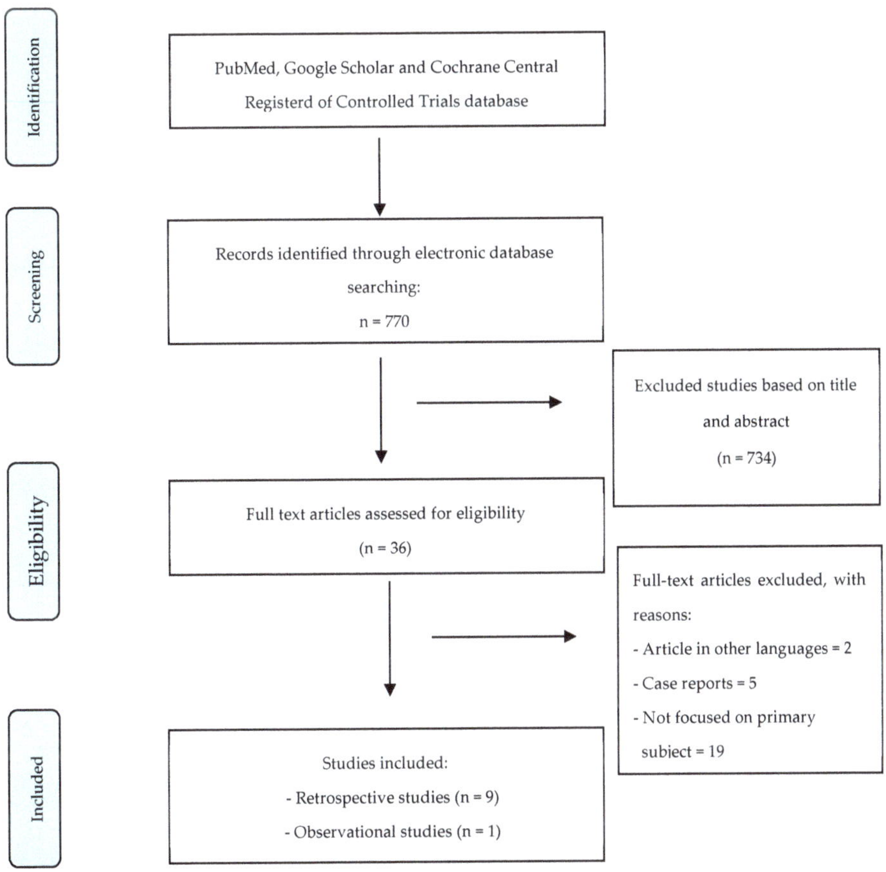


**Figure 1.** PRISMA flow diagram for systematic research and selection of studies included in the review.

The inclusion criteria in the selection of the studies were as follows:

- Hepatic bleeding from a traumatic cause, either blunt or penetrating;
- Endovascular treatment used alone or in combination with surgical procedures to treat only hepatic injuries;
- Description of the HD status of the patient, with a focus on articles where unstable patients were treated;
- Evaluation of the outcomes after embolization.

The following exclusion criteria were included:

- Case reports;
- Studies in which embolization for the treatment of liver bleeding was used in stable patients;

- Studies in which the population was pediatric;
- Studies where the endovascular treatment was used to treat non-traumatic liver injuries.

### 2.1. Outcomes

The primary outcomes evaluated included the clinical success rate, all-cause mortality and overall morbidity post-procedure among the HD unstable liver trauma patients treated with embolization. The common complications after endovascular treatment were considered, such as liver abscess/biloma formation, bile leak, gallbladder necrosis/acute cholecystitis, peritonitis and abdominal compartment syndrome. Moreover, the AAST classification was investigated to relate the presence of a correlation between the severity of the liver injury and the HD status of the patients.

### 2.2. Data Extraction

Two reviewers (F.C. and F.G.) screened titles first individually and then together to choose the appropriate articles. All of the data needed for the studies were extracted and tabulated after an in-depth reading process; the results are presented using descriptive statistics, and dichotomous and continuous variables are reported as absolute numbers, means, percentages, ranges and ratios as appropriate.

## 3. Results

According to the inclusion and exclusion criteria, initially, a total of 770 references were identified. The first evaluation of the title and abstract allowed us to exclude a total of 734 references. The remaining 36 articles were further considered for inclusion in the review and evaluated in the full-article review step. A total of 18 of them were excluded because they did not focus on the primary subject, 5 of them were excluded because they were case reports and 2 of them were excluded because they were not written in the English language. Finally, a total of 10 studies were included in the review [9–18]. Almost all of them were retrospective studies and only one was an observational study. Table 1 summarizes the main characteristics of the studies included and the number and demographic details of the enrolled patients.

**Table 1.** General characteristics of the studies included in the review.

| Authors | Year | Study Type | Total Patients | M/F Ratio | Mean Age | Total Primary Embolization in Unstable Patients | % Grade Trauma (AAST) |
|---|---|---|---|---|---|---|---|
| Tamura S et al. [9] | 2021 | RT | 92 | 3.7/1 | 29.5 | 59 | Grade III (58%)<br>Grade IV (34%)<br>Grade V (8%) |
| Aoki M et al. [10] | 2021 | RT | 224 | 1.5/1 | 55 | 57 | Grade III (40%)<br>Grade IV (18%)<br>Grade V (5%) |
| Alnumay A et al. [11] | 2021 | RT | 49 | 4/1 | 44 | 5 | Not available |
| Inukai K et al. [12] | 2018 | RT | 23 | 1/1 | 32.3 | 10 | Grade IV (80%)<br>Grade V (20%) |
| Otsuka et al. [13] | 2017 | OB | 16 | 3/1 | 46 | 5 | Grade III (40%)<br>Grade IV (20%)<br>Grade V (40%) |
| Ogura et al. [14] | 2014 | RT | 7 | 3/1 | 63.5 | 3 | Grade II (33%)<br>Grade IV (34%)<br>Grade V (33%) |
| Mitsusada M et al. [15] | 2013 | RT | 29 | 2.2/1 | 38.5 | 8 | Not available |
| Di Saverio S et al. [16] | 2012 | RT | 34 | 1.5/1 | 42 | 10 | Not available |
| Misselbeck TS et al. [17] | 2009 | RT | 21 | N/A | N/A | 11 | Not available |
| Monnin et al. [18] | 2007 | RT | 12 | N/A | 35 | 3 | Grade IV (100%) |

### 3.1. Patient Demographics

We collected pooled data on 507 HD unstable liver trauma patients from 10 separate articles selected according to the inclusion and exclusion criteria; of these 507 patients, only 171 underwent a primary embolization treatment. Patients included in the studies had predominantly severe liver trauma. The American Association for the Surgery of Trauma (AAST) injury grade rate of the different studies is reported in Table 1; however, only six articles reported the AAST grade exact number of HD unstable trauma patients [19].

### 3.2. Hemodynamic Status

One of the main focus points of this review concerns the HD status of the patients and its definition; the different definitions available for the HD status of the patients among the 11 studies are summarized in Table 2. There were many differences between single studies in the definition of HD unstable/transient responder patients. Only one article identified HD unstable liver trauma patients using the Shock Index (SI), defined by the ratio of the heart rate (HR) to the systolic blood pressure (sBP) [9]. The majority of articles used the sBP but with different values. Aoki et al. defined unstable patients as those who had an sBP < 90 mmHg upon hospital arrival and received blood transfusion within the first 24 h after arrival [10]. In the same way, Otsuka et al. considered unstable patients those who displayed persistent hypotension with an sBP < 90 mmHg following primary resuscitation and Ogura et al. considered the cut-off of an sBP maintained at 70 mmHg. The first study considered stabilized patients as those who responded to resuscitative therapy and the second two, instead, considered HD unstable patients stabilized with resuscitative endovascular balloon occlusion of the aorta (REBOA) [13,14]. Inukai et al. and Mitsusada et al. considered HD unstable patients first as those that reached an sBP ≥ 90 mmHg for even a second after rapid fluid infusion or blood transfusion, and second as those with a value of sBP ≥ 80 mmHg after resuscitative therapy [12–15].

**Table 2.** Different definitions of hemodynamic stability and instability.

| Authors | Year | Definition of Stable Patient | Definition of Unstable Patient |
|---|---|---|---|
| Tamura S et al. [9] | 2021 | All trauma patients responding to initial standard infusion therapy (crystalloid, albumin and blood transfusion) | SI > 1, despite initial infusion therapy |
| Aoki M et al. [10] | 2021 | sBP ≥ 90 mmHg upon hospital arrival | sBP < 90 mmHg upon hospital arrival and received blood transfusion within the first 24 h after arrival |
| Alnumay A et al. [11] | 2021 | Not available | Not available |
| Inukai K et al. [12] | 2018 | sBP ≥ 90 mmHg after initial fluid treatment | sBP ≥ 90 mmHg for even a second and therefore required rapid fluid infusion or blood transfusion |
| Otsuka et al. [13] | 2017 | sBP ≥ 90 mmHg after initial fluid treatment | sBP < 90 mmHg without improvement following primary resuscitation |
| Ogura et al. [14] | 2014 | Not available | sBP maintained at 70 mm Hg or greater during deflation of the balloon (REBOA) |
| Mitsusada M et al. [15] | 2013 | Not available | sBP ≥ 80 mmHg after resuscitative therapy |
| Di Saverio S et al. [16] | 2012 | Not available | Not available |
| Misselbeck TS et al. [17] | 2009 | At admission, sBP was ≥ 90 mm Hg and intravenous fluid requirements did not exceed 2 L. | Not available |
| Monnin et al. [18] | 2007 | Patients who were hemodynamically stable or stabilized by low or moderate resuscitation. | Patients with hemorrhagic shock improved or stabilized after resuscitative treatment. |

### 3.3. Mortality and Morbidity

All of the outcome measures were evaluated and are reported in Table 3. The number of patients with failure of the arterial embolization procedure were reported only in five studies, with a total number of four patients and a rate of 2,33%. Moreover, in only four studies, there was no report of mortality in HD liver trauma patients; a total average of 9.3% of mortality with a range between 3.2 and 36% was reported. The most frequent cause of mortality was not due to liver injury, but it was related to a concomitant severe head trauma with very low grade on the Glasgow Coma Scale (GCS) at admission.

**Table 3.** Rate and type of mortality and morbidity reported in individual studies.

| Authors | Year | Total Number of Embolized Patients *N* | Mortality *N* (%) | AE Failure *N* (%) | Post-AE Complications *N* (%) |
|---|---|---|---|---|---|
| Tamura S et al. [9] | 2021 | 59 | 3 (3.2) | 2 (2.1) | 29 (31.5) |
| Aoki M et al. [10] | 2021 | 57 | 7 (12) | Not available | 9 (15.7) |
| Alnumay A et al. [11] | 2021 | 5 | Not available | Not available | Not available |
| Inukai K et al. [12] | 2018 | 10 | 1 (10) | 0 | 5 (50) |
| Otsuka et al. [13] | 2017 | 5 | Not available | 1 (20) | 4 (80) |
| Ogura et al. [14] | 2014 | 3 | 1 (33) | Not available | Not available |
| Mitsusada M et al. [15] | 2013 | 8 | 0 | 0 | 3 (37.5) |
| Di Saverio S et al. [16] | 2012 | 10 | Not available | Not available | Not available |
| Misselbeck TS et al. [17] | 2009 | 11 | 4 (36) | 1 (9) | 9 (81) |
| Monnin et al. [18] | 2007 | 3 | N/A | N/A | N/A |
| TOTAL | | 171 | 16 (9.35) | 4 (2.33) | 59 (34.5) |

Only in four studies was it not possible to determine the number of complications related to the embolization procedure (Table 4). The average complication rate was 34.5%, with a range between 15.7% and 80%. The most common complication reported was liver abscess/biloma with an incidence of 12.8% and a range between 5.26 and 36%. Bile leakage was reported with a mean incidence of 3% and a range between 3% and 37.5%. Gallbladder necrosis was reported in seven studies with a mean incidence of 5.3% and a range between 1% and 66%. Peritonitis was reported with a mean incidence of 6.4% and a range between 5.2 and 54%. Finally, abdominal compartment syndrome complication was reported in only six studies and occurred with a mean incidence of 1.16% and a range between 1.16% and 20%. Hepatic ischemia was not evaluated as a complication because it is a well-known outcome due to the embolization procedure. No study took into consideration the individualized complication rate according to the embolic agent used.

**Table 4.** Rate and type of complications reported in individual studies.

| Authors | Year | Total Number of Embolized Patients *N* | Liver Abscess/Biloma *N* (%) | Bile Leakage *N* (%) | Gallbladder Necrosis/Cholecystitis *N* (%) | Peritonitis *N* (%) | Abdominal Compartment Syndrome *N* (%) |
|---|---|---|---|---|---|---|---|
| Tamura S et al. [9] | 2021 | 59 | 13 (14.1) | 0 | 1 (1.08) | 0 | 0 |
| Aoki M et al. [10] | 2021 | 57 | 3 (5.26) | 0 | 1 (1.7) | 3 (5.2) | Not available |
| Alnumay A et al. [11] | 2021 | 5 | Not available | Not available | Not available | Not available | Not available |
| Inukai K et al. [12] | 2018 | 10 | 2 (20) | 1 (10) | 0 | 0 | 2 (20) |

**Table 4.** *Cont.*

| Authors | Year | Total Number of Embolized Patients *N* | Liver Abscess/Biloma *N* (%) | Bile Leakage *N* (%) | Gallbladder Necrosis/Cholecystitis *N* (%) | Peritonitis *N* (%) | Abdominal Compartment Syndrome *N* (%) |
|---|---|---|---|---|---|---|---|
| Otsuka et al. [13] | 2017 | 5 | 0 | 0 | 1 (20) | 2 (40) | 0 |
| Ogura et al. [14] | 2014 | 3 | Not available | Not available | Not available | Not available | Not available |
| Mitsusada M et al. [15] | 2013 | 8 | 0 | 3 (37.5) | 0 | 0 | 0 |
| Di Saverio S et al. [16] | 2012 | 10 | Not available | Not available | Not available | Not available | Not available |
| Misselbeck TS et al. [17] | 2009 | 11 | 4 (36) | 1 (9) | 6 (66) | 6 (54) | 0 |
| Monnin et al. [18] | 2007 | 3 | Not available | Not available | Not available | Not available | Not available |
| TOTAL | | 171 | 22 (12.8) | 5 (3) | 9 (5.3) | 11 (6.4) | 2 (1.16) |

## 4. Discussion

WSES guidelines recommend TAE as the first-line therapy in HD stable patients with blunt or penetrating liver trauma; on the other hand, operative management (OM) (level of evidence I) is recommended in HD unstable patients with no indication for NOM [8]. To date, there are no comparative studies of TAE and OM in HD unstable liver trauma patients.

One of the main issues of this review is the definition of unstable patients, where our review found notable heterogeneity in the definition between the individual studies; the majority of the studies considered in our review define unstable patients as those who can benefit from TAE and those who initially respond to massive fluid and blood resuscitation, according to WSES guidelines, are categorized as transient responder patients. These patients could be stable enough to undergo a CT scan and can also be managed non-surgically. Trauma protocols of every hospital are based on the Advanced Trauma Life Support (ATLS) program, created by the American College of Surgeons Committee on Trauma. In the ATLS program, the definition of shock state is related to the evaluation of sBP, HR and base deficit (BD); however, the cut-off points of these vital signs have been disputed by some authors [20]. A recent systematic review points out that HD stability is the most important factor in the assessment of trauma patients; however, no consensus on the definition of HD stability between individual trauma centers has been demonstrated in the literature, pointing out that only a limited number of patients can be classified into the current ATLS shock classification [1]. However, further high-quality studies are needed to confirm this statement and a specific indication about the treatment of this kind of patient should be addressed more extensively by new guideline revisions.

A recent observational study demonstrated a >50% change in the management of HD unstable trauma patients subjected to a prior contrast-enhanced computed tomography (CT) scan. CT scans may have a role in detecting and managing such patients appropriately; however, in this paper, there is no clear definition of HD instability and whether the patients are partial responders or not to the initial resuscitative management [21].

Our review demonstrates a good outcome in partially responding unstable patients treated with TAE and NOM in institutions where there is 24 h availability of an IR team that could perform a prompt embolization treatment. Tamura et al. demonstrated a similar outcome in HD unstable liver trauma patients (who initially responded to infusion therapy) treated with TAE and NOM as compared to stable liver trauma patients treated with NOM. TAE for HD unstable patients with liver injury does not increase the mortality rates (6% in this series compared to 3–8% of an observational study) [22]. Moreover, the TAE group demonstrates fewer massive transfusions and shorter intensive care unit (ICU) stays than the OM group. However, in a multivariate analysis, the only predictor of ICU stay and massive transfusion was the initial HD status, and thus, they may not be related to treatment [9].

A recent systematic review and meta-analysis demonstrated a good clinical success rate (91%), bleeding resolution and the absence of further intervention, and a low mortality rate (7%) due to NOM in solid organ trauma HD unstable patients; moreover, one of the main inclusion criteria for TAE in HD unstable patients is an initial response to the initial resuscitative management that allows the target blood pressure to reached that is required to access the angiographic suite and perform the procedure [23]

One of the most important factors in determining the success rate of TAE in unstable patients depends on the time elapsed from CT diagnosis and the endovascular procedure. A cohort study reported that the presence of a pathway where CT study and TAE were performed within 30 min in unstable patients who were either complete or partial transient responders to the resuscitative protocol, as well as in patients who were in a shock state upon initial admission, resulted in a decreased rate of OM with a similar mortality rate [24]. However, it must be emphasized that in these management options, there should be rapid availability of an operating team if the patients' conditions deteriorate. On the other hand, in trauma centers where IR facilities were not promptly available, only 6% of the HD unstable patients underwent the TAE procedure [25].

Hemorrhage control is time-critical, emphasized by the data demonstrating that delays in operative intervention in patients with significant abdominal injuries caused a 1% higher mortality risk for every 3 min of delay in reaching the operating room [26]. Damage control surgery in liver trauma is based on the surgical dogma "Push, Pack and Pringle", which summarizes the main surgical maneuvers that surgeons must perform to limit bleeding. Most venous bleeding could be controlled by a liver packing procedure; however, arterial injury could continue to produce bleeding, and TAE, associated with packing, may rule out hemorrhage control [27]. For this reason, the choice of which patients could benefit from an immediate operative management versus angiographic study is critical, especially with these partial responder unstable patients where time is everything; the development of hybrid operating rooms, which allow surgeons to perform multiple bleeding control procedures in the same location, eliminating the need to move patients back and forth between rows, showed potential reductions in mortality and procedure time. The RAPTOR study demonstrated a significant reduction in treatment time, with about 18% of patients requiring an emergent percutaneous procedural intervention added to open surgery and showing a clear benefit for survival (42% RAPTOR era vs. 22% pre-RAPTOR era) in a hybrid suite. However, this study postulated that the cost associated with a hybrid suite, where an advanced angiography system is available, remains prohibitive for many centers [28,29]. Another cheaper solution could be the use of a mobile C-arm in an operating room equipped with a carbon-fiber fluoroscopic table [11].

The resuscitative endovascular balloon occlusion of the aorta (REBOA) could be another useful strategy in HD unstable patients that require direct OM; however, the evidence base on its use in liver trauma patients is weak and there is no clear indication on the time and zone of balloon inflation. Its use in HD unstable patients with multiple severe torso trauma refractory undergoing initial infusion therapy has been reported to improve prognosis [14].

To the best of our knowledge, this is one of the first systematic reviews that summarizes patient outcomes regarding TAE in HD unstable/transient responder liver trauma patients. Nevertheless, there are some limitations to this study that should be noted. First, the total sample size was low, which lowered the validity of the present results and indicates that large-scale studies on this topic, especially prospective studies, are needed. Second, the majority of the included studies are retrospective or observational studies. Therefore, high-quality trials to explore the efficacy and safety of angioembolization in this setting are needed. Finally, we did not study the selection criteria of patients for angioembolization in this setting.

## 5. Conclusions

IR is a fundament of trauma patients' care and management; one of the greatest limitations of endovascular treatment is represented by being classified as a NOM. TAE should be compared to a surgical operation, with its well-known risks and complications, and it should be no longer counted as NOM but rather as OM or differentiated by creating a new section management known as endovascular treatment. To date, the role of IR in the management and treatment of patients with severe liver trauma has been well known; our review demonstrated a very good outcome in HD unstable/transient responder patients treated with TAE. However, there still remains much debate about the definition of unstable patients and transient responder patients to resuscitative treatment because these are borderline situations in which it is very difficult to identify clear parameters, both clinical and biochemical. Using TAE in unstable/transient responder liver trauma patients is feasible, but more prospective studies, even better if they are multicentric, are needed to standardize the treatment and also to clear the fog that exists regarding the definition of the HD status of patients.

**Author Contributions:** Conceptualization, F.C. and F.G.; methodology, F.C., A.B. and M.G.; validation, P.M., M.G. and R.N.; formal analysis, F.C.; investigation, F.C.; data curation, F.C. and F.G; writing—original draft preparation, F.C., M.G., A.M.I. and R.N.; writing—review and editing, M.G., A.I., A.C. and R.N.; supervision, M.G. and R.N. All authors have read and agreed to the published version of the manuscript.

**Funding:** This research received no external funding.

**Institutional Review Board Statement:** This study does not require ethical approval.

**Informed Consent Statement:** Not applicable.

**Data Availability Statement:** No new data were created or analyzed in this study. Data sharing is not applicable to this article.

**Conflicts of Interest:** The authors declare no conflicts of interest.

## References

1. Loggers, S.A.I.; Koedam, T.W.A.; Giannakopoulos, G.F.; Vandewalle, E.; Erwteman, M.; Zuidema, W.P. Definition of hemodynamic stability in blunt trauma patients: A systematic review and assessment amongst Dutch trauma team members. *Eur. J. Trauma Emerg. Surg.* **2017**, *43*, 823–833. [CrossRef]
2. Matsushima, K.; Piccinini, A.; Schellenberg, M.; Cheng, V.; Heindel, P.; Strumwasser, A.; Benjamin, E.; Inaba, K.; Demetriades, D. Effect of door-to-angioembolization time on mortality in pelvic fracture: Every hour of delay counts. *J. Trauma Acute Care Surg.* **2018**, *84*, 685–692. [CrossRef]
3. American College of Surgeons Committee on Trauma. Resources for Optimal Care of the Injured Patient. 2022. Available online: https://www.facs.org/quality-programs/trauma/quality/verification-review-and-consultation-program/standards/ (accessed on 2 November 2022).
4. Mathew, J.K.; Fitzgerald, M.C. Damage Control Interventional Radiology (DCIR): Evolving Value of Interventional Radiology in Trauma. *Cardiovasc. Interv. Radiol.* **2022**, *45*, 1757–1758. [CrossRef]
5. Clements, W.; Koukounaras, J.; Joseph, T. Reply to "Damage Control Interventional Radiology (DCIR): Evolving Value of In-terventional Radiology in Trauma". *Cardiovasc. Interv. Radiol.* **2022**, *45*, 1759–1761. [CrossRef] [PubMed]
6. Segalini, E.; Morello, A.; Leati, G.; Di Saverio, S.; Aseni, P. Primary angioembolization in liver trauma: Major hepatic necrosis as a severe complication of a minimally invasive treatment-a narrative review. *Updates Surg.* **2022**, *74*, 1511–1519. [CrossRef]
7. Roberts, R.; Sheth, R.A. Hepatic Trauma. *Ann. Transl. Med.* **2021**, *9*, 1195. [CrossRef]
8. Coccolini, F.; Panel, T.W.E.; Coimbra, R.; Ordonez, C.; Kluger, Y.; Vega, F.; Moore, E.E.; Biffl, W.; Peitzman, A.; Horer, T.; et al. Liver trauma: WSES 2020 guidelines. *World J. Emerg. Surg.* **2020**, *15*, 24. [CrossRef] [PubMed]
9. Tamura, S.; Maruhashi, T.; Kashimi, F.; Kurihara, Y.; Masuda, T.; Hanajima, T.; Kataoka, Y.; Asari, Y. Transcatheter arterial embolization for severe blunt liver injury in hemodynamically unstable patients: A 15-year retrospective study. *Scand. J. Trauma Resusc. Emerg. Med.* **2021**, *29*, 66. [CrossRef] [PubMed]
10. Aoki, M.; Abe, T.; Hagiwara, S.; Saitoh, D.; Oshima, K. Embolization versus Surgery for Stabilized Patients with Solid Organ Injury. *J. Vasc. Interv. Radiol.* **2021**, *32*, 1150–1155.e5. [CrossRef]
11. Alnumay, A.; Caminsky, N.; Eustache, J.H.; Valenti, D.; Beckett, A.N.; Deckelbaum, D.; Fata, P.; Khwaja, K.; Razek, T.; McKendy, K.M.; et al. Feasibility of intraoperative angioembolization for trauma patients using C-arm digital subtraction angiography. *Eur. J. Trauma Emerg. Surg.* **2022**, *48*, 315–319. [CrossRef]

12. Inukai, K.; Uehara, S.; Furuta, Y.; Miura, M. Nonoperative management of blunt liver injury in hemodynamically stable versus unstable patients: A retrospective study. *Emerg. Radiol.* **2018**, *25*, 647–652. [CrossRef]
13. Otsuka, H.; Sato, T.; Sakurai, K.; Aoki, H.; Yamagiwa, T.; Iizuka, S.; Inokuchi, S. Use of interventional radiology as initial hemorrhage control to improve outcomes for potentially lethal multiple blunt injuries. *Injury* **2018**, *49*, 226–229. [CrossRef] [PubMed]
14. Ogura, T.; Lefor, A.T.; Nakano, M.; Izawa, Y.; Morita, H. Nonoperative management of hemodynamically unstable abdominal trauma patients with angioembolization and resuscitative endovascular balloon occlusion of the aorta. *J. Trauma Acute Care Surg.* **2015**, *78*, 132–135. [CrossRef]
15. Mitsusada, M.; Nakajima, Y.; Shirokawa, M.; Takeda, T.; Honda, H. Non-operative management of blunt liver injury: A new protocol for selected hemodynamically unstable patients under hypotensive resuscitation. *J. Hepatobiliary Pancreat. Sci.* **2014**, *21*, 205–211. [CrossRef]
16. Di Saverio, S.; Catena, F.; Filicori, F.; Ansaloni, L.; Coccolini, F.; Keutgen, X.M.; Giugni, A.; Coniglio, C.; Biscardi, A.; Cavallo, P.; et al. Predictive factors of morbidity and mortality in grade IV and V liver trauma undergoing perihepatic packing: Single institution 14 years experience at European trauma centre. *Injury* **2012**, *43*, 1347–1354. [CrossRef]
17. Misselbeck, T.S.; Teicher, E.J.; Cipolle, M.D.; Pasquale, M.D.; Shah, K.T.; Dangleben, D.A.; Badellino, M.M. Hepatic angioembolization in trauma patients: Indications and complications. *J. Trauma* **2009**, *67*, 769–773. [CrossRef]
18. Monnin, V.; Sengel, C.; Thony, F.; Bricault, I.; Voirin, D.; Letoublon, C.; Broux, C.; Ferretti, G. Place of arterial embolization in severe blunt hepatic trauma: A multidisciplinary approach. *Cardiovasc. Interv. Radiol.* **2008**, *31*, 875–882. [CrossRef] [PubMed]
19. Moore, E.E.; Cogbill, T.H.; Jurkovich, G.J.; Shackford, S.R.; Malangoni, M.A.; Champion, H.R. Organ injury scaling Spleen and liver (1994 revision). *J. Trauma* **1995**, *38*, 323–324. [CrossRef]
20. American College of Surgeons. *Advanced Trauma Life Support for Doctors*, 8th ed.; American College of Surgeons: Chicago, IL, USA, 2008.
21. Kim, Y.J.; Kim, J.S.; Cho, S.H.; Bae, J.I.; Sohn, C.H.; Lee, Y.S.; Lee, J.H.; Lim, K.S.; Kim, W.Y. Characteristics of computed tomography in hemodynamically unstable blunt trauma patients: Experience at a tertiary care center. *Medicine* **2017**, *96*, e9168. [CrossRef]
22. Gaski, I.A.; Skattum, J.; Brooks, A.; Koyama, T.; Eken, T.; Naess, P.A.; Gaarder, C. Decreased mortality, laparotomy, and embolization rates for liver injuries during a 13-year period in a major Scandinavian trauma center. *Trauma Surg. Acute Care Open* **2018**, *3*, e000205. [CrossRef]
23. Tan, T.; Luo, Y.; Hu, J.; Li, F.; Fu, Y. Nonoperative management with angioembolization for blunt abdominal solid organ trauma in hemodynamically unstable patients: A systematic review and meta-analysis. *Eur. J. Trauma Emerg. Surg.* **2022**, *49*, 1751–1761. [CrossRef] [PubMed]
24. Gaarder, C.; Naess, P.A.; Eken, T.; Skaga, N.O.; Pillgram-Larsen, J.; Klow, N.E.; Buanes, T. Liver injuries--improved results with a formal protocol including angiography. *Injury* **2007**, *38*, 1075–1083. [CrossRef] [PubMed]
25. Bertens, K.A.; Vogt, K.N.; Hernandez-Alejandro, R.; Gray, D.K. Non-operative management of blunt hepatic trauma: Does angioembolization have a major impact? *Eur. J. Trauma Emerg. Surg.* **2014**, *41*, 81–86. [CrossRef] [PubMed]
26. Clarke, J.R.; Trooskin, S.Z.; Doshi, P.J.; Greenwald, L.; Mode, C.J. Time to laparotomy for intra-abdominal bleeding from trauma does affect survival for delays up to 90 min. *J. Trauma* **2002**, *52*, 420–425. [PubMed]
27. Kanani, A.; Sandve, K.O.; Søreide, K. Management of severe liver injuries: Push, pack, pringle—And plug! *Scand. J. Trauma, Resusc. Emerg. Med.* **2021**, *29*, 93. [CrossRef] [PubMed]
28. Carver, D.; Kirkpatrick, A.W.; D'Amours, S.; Hameed, S.M.; Beveridge, J.; Ball, C.G. A Prospective Evaluation of the Utility of a Hybrid. Operating Suite for Severely Injured Patients: Overstated or Underutilized? *Ann. Surg.* **2020**, *271*, 958–961. [CrossRef]
29. Kirkpatrick, A.W.; Vis, C.; Dubé, M.; Biesbroek, S.; Ball, C.G.; Laberge, J.; Shultz, J.; Rea, K.; Sadler, D.; Holcomb, J.B.; et al. The evolution of a purpose designed hybrid trauma operating room from the trauma service perspective: The RAPTOR (Resuscitation with Angiography Percutaneous Treatments and Operative Resuscitations). *Injury* **2014**, *45*, 1413–1421. [CrossRef]

Journal of *Personalized Medicine*

MDPI

*Review*

# Irreversible Electroporation (IRE) for Prostate Cancer (PCa) Treatment: The State of the Art

**Eliodoro Faiella, Domiziana Santucci, Daniele Vertulli *, Elva Vergantino, Federica Vaccarino, Gloria Perillo, Bruno Beomonte Zobel and Rosario Francesco Grasso**

Department of Radiology, Policlinico "Campus Bio-medico", Via Alvaro del Portillo, 200-00128 Rome, Italy; e.faiella@policlinicocampus.it (E.F.); d.santucci@policlinicocampus.it (D.S.); elva.vergantino@unicampus.it (E.V.); federica.vaccarino@unicampus.it (F.V.); gloria.perillo@unicampus.it (G.P.); b.zobel@policlinicocampus.it (B.B.Z.); r.grasso@policlinicocampus.it (R.F.G.)

* Correspondence: daniele.vertulli@unicampus.it

**Abstract:** We evaluated the most recent research from 2000 to 2023 in order to deeply investigate the applications of PCa IRE, first exploring its usage with primary intent and then salvage intent. Finally, we discuss the differences with other focal PCa treatments. In the case of primary-intent IRE, the in-field recurrence is quite low (ranges from 0% to 33%). Urinary continence after the treatment remains high (>86%). Due to several different patients in the studies, the preserved potency varied quite a lot (59–100%). Regarding complications, the highest occurrence rates are for those of Grades I and II (20–77% and 0–29%, respectively). Grade III complications represent less than 7%. Regarding the specific oncological outcomes, both PCa-specific survival and overall survival are 100%. Metastasis-free survival is 99.6%. In a long-term study, the Kaplan–Meier FFS rates reported are 91% at 3 years, 84% at 5 years, and 69% at 8 years. In the single study with salvage-intent IRE, the in-field recurrence was 7%. Urinary continence was still high (93%), but preserved potency was significantly lower than primary-intent IRE patients (23%). In addition, Grade III complications were slightly higher (10.8%). In conclusion, in males with localized low–intermediate-risk prostate cancer, IRE had an excellent safety profile and might have positive results for sexual and urinary function.

**Keywords:** irreversible electroporation; prostate cancer; cancers treatments; interventional radiology; IRE

## 1. Introduction

In the last decades, due to widespread screening practices, prostate cancer (PCa) has recently been identified at earlier stages. Although drastic procedures, such as radical prostatectomy (RP) and external beam radiation therapy (EBRT), are considered as the standard treatments for patients with low to intermediate risk [1], a currently growing interest about overtreatment has prompted researchers to work towards investigating less invasive alternatives. Partial prostate ablation, which sits in the midst of active surveillance and radical treatments, attempts to treat PCa while preserving the gland tissue portion necessary to maintain genitourinary function [2].

Multiparametric magnetic resonance imaging (mpMRI) has demonstrated to be extremely accurate both for the localization of PCa lesions and the guiding of target lesion biopsy [3,4]. The correct identification of a lesion is necessary before ablation treatment. Additionally, the creation of ablative technology has made it possible for us to remove tumor foci while protecting adjacent tissue.

Irreversible electroporation (IRE) stands at the forefront of emerging ablative techniques, and is currently under thorough investigation within the medical community. For urologists seeking to incorporate these novel technologies into their practice, a comprehensive understanding of the scientific foundations is imperative. Unlike conventional treatment modalities that rely on non-selective thermal destruction, IRE represents a paradigm shift by employing a non-thermal approach, strategically designed to annihilate targeted cells while preserving vital structures. The distinctive feature of IRE lies in its utilization of brief yet potent electrical fields, harnessing their capacity to puncture cell membranes permanently and lethally. This precise disruption of cellular membranes results in the creation of nanopores and a consequential modification of cell membrane permeability. The cumulative effect of these processes induces apoptosis, providing a unique mechanism for cell death that distinguishes IRE from other ablative techniques. It is noteworthy that despite being primarily characterized as a non-thermal mechanism, recent studies, particularly in porcine models, have elucidated the generation of heat during the IRE process. This intriguing revelation adds a layer of complexity to the understanding of IRE, suggesting that the interplay between non-thermal and thermal effects may contribute to the overall efficacy of the treatment. As researchers delve deeper into the intricacies of IRE, exploring its mechanisms at the cellular and molecular levels, the potential applications and nuances of this technology become increasingly apparent. The ability to selectively target cells for destruction without causing collateral damage to surrounding structures holds great promise for various medical fields, especially in the realm of urology. The ongoing exploration of IRE represents a pioneering venture into the realm of focused ablative techniques. Its non-thermal methodology, coupled with the recent insights into heat generation, adds a layer of sophistication to its application. Urologists and radiologists navigating this landscape of innovation must continue to unravel the complexities of IRE, paving the way for its judicious and effective integration into clinical practice [5].

Providing sharp ablation zone margins is one of IRE's benefits. It is generally agreed that only a few cell layers separate the reversibly electroporated area from the irreversibly electroporated area. In contrast, there are no transition zones like in thermal- or radiation-based ablation procedures. Real-time monitoring is an additional advantage. Both during and after the treatment, it is possible to partially view the treatment volume. Possible visualization techniques include MRI, CT, and ultrasound [6].

In this review, we critically evaluate the most recent researches in order to deeply investigate the PCa IRE applications, first exploring its primary-intent usage and then its salvage-intent usage. Finally, we discuss the differences with other focal PCa treatments.

## 2. Materials and Methods

A literature search was performed using the Medical Literature Analysis and Retrieval System Online (MEDLINE), the Excerpta Medica dataBASE (EMBASE), PubMed, and Google Scholar. The following terms were entered into the search algorithm to identify articles: 'prostate irreversible electroporation', 'irreversible electroporation'. The search was limited to articles in English published between 2000 and 2023. The authors reviewed the retrieved articles by using a PRISMA flowchart (Figure 1), and the references of the retrieved articles were used when relevant.

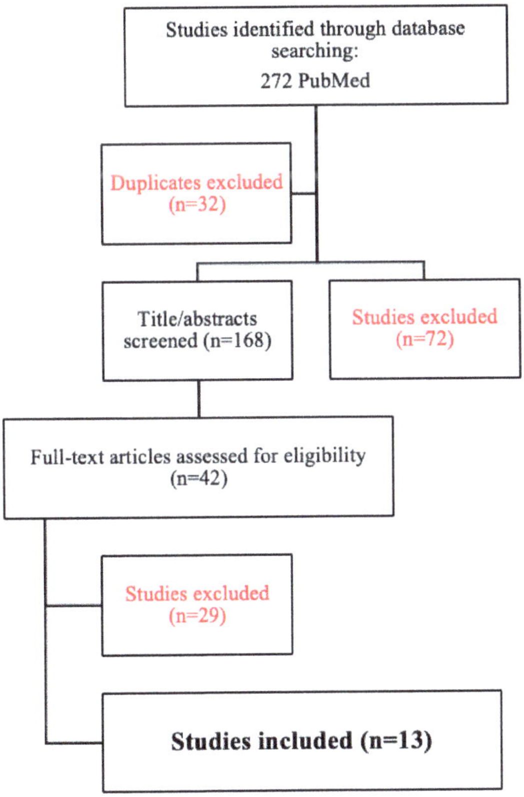


**Figure 1.** PRISMA (preferred reporting items for systematic reviews and meta-analysis) 2009 flowchart for study search and selection. Red color data have been excluded because of no utility for this study or other reasons.

## 3. Results

A total of 13 studies were included in this review, which were divided according to the modality of the IRE (primary-intent and salvage-intent after RT). Finally we included a single study which reported the differences between focal and diffuse IRE. In particular, 12 studies were in a primary-intent IRE setting, and 1 was in a salvage-intent setting.

See Table 1 for the complete overview of the studies.

**Table 1.** Overview of characteristics, outcomes, and complications of studies about IRE treatment.

| Year | First Author | Intent | Patients | PSA (Mean), Age (Mean) | Outcomes | Complications |
|---|---|---|---|---|---|---|
| 2010 | Onik [7] | Primary | 16 | 3–7; 40–78 | No in-field recurrence<br>100% continence<br>100% preserved potency | Not reported |
| 2014 | Neal [8] | Primary | 2 | 4.5; 61 | No in-field recurrence | Not reported |
| 2014 | Valerio [9] | Primary | 19 | 7.5; 60 | In-field recurrence: 33%<br>100% continence<br>95% preserved potency | Grade I: 12 (35%)<br>Grade II: 10 (29%)<br>Grade III: 0 |
| 2016 | Ting [10] | Primary | 32 | 6; 67 | No in-field recurrence<br>100% continence<br>100% preserved potency | Grade I: 5 (20%)<br>Grade II: 0<br>Grade III: 1 (4%) |

**Table 1.** *Cont.*

| Year | First Author | Intent | Patients | PSA (Mean), Age (Mean) | Outcomes | Complications |
|---|---|---|---|---|---|---|
| 2016 | Murray [11] | Primary | 25 | 4.5; 63.2 | In-field recurrence: 16%<br>100% continence<br>95% preserved potency | Grade I: 6 (22%)<br>Grade II: 7 (29%)<br>Grade III: 1 (7%) |
| 2018 | Scheltema [12] | Primary | 50 | 5.9; 67 | In-field recurrence: 29.5%<br>98% continence (same in RP)<br>69% preserved potency (68% in RP) | Grade. . . IRE vs. RP<br>Grade I: 11 (22) vs. 9 (16%)<br>Grade II: 7 (13.7%) vs. 5 (9%)<br>Grade III: 0 vs. 0 |
| 2018 | Van den Bos [13] | Primary | 63 | 6; 67 | In-field recurrence: 16%<br>100% continence<br>77% preserved potency | Grade I: 15 (24%)<br>Grade II: 7 (11%)<br>Grade III: 0 |
| 2019 | Collettini [14] | Primary | 30 | 8.65; 65.5 | In-field recurrence: 17.9%<br>86.2% continence (vs. 90% at baseline)<br>79.3% preserved potency (vs. 83.3% at baseline) | Grade I: 6 (20%)<br>Grade II: 3 (10%)<br>Grade III: 1 (3.3%) |
| 2020 | Blazevski [15] | Primary | 123 | 5.7; 68 | In-field recurrence: 2.7–9.8%<br>98.8% continence<br>76% preserved potency<br>FFS at three years: 99%<br>Overall survival: 100% | Not reported |
| 2021 | Blazevski [16] | Primary | 50 | 6.25; 68 | In-field recurrence: 2.5%<br>98% continence<br>59% preserved potency (vs. 65% at baseline) | Grade I: 10 (20%)<br>Grade II: 9 (18%)<br>Grade III: 0 |
| 2022 | De la Rosette [17] | Primary (local vs. diffuse IRE) | 51 | 5.93; 64 | Higher IEEF-5 and EPIC scores at 3 months follow up in focal IRE than diffuse IRE<br>6 month biopsy with residual PCa: 18.8% vs. 13.2% (no significance) | Grades. . . focal vs. diffuse<br>Grade I: 23 (77%) vs. 27 (79%)<br>Grade II: 6 (20%) vs. 7 (21%)<br>Grade III: 9 (3.3%) vs. 0 |
| 2023 | Geboers [18] | Salvage | 74 | 5.4; 69 | In-field recurrence: 7%<br>93% continence<br>23% preserved potency | Grade I-II: 6 (8.1%)<br>Grade III: 8 (10.8%) |
| 2023 | Scheltema [19] | Primary | 229 | 5.9; 68 | In-field recurrence: 24%<br>98–99% continence<br>71% preserved potency (vs. 58% at baseline)<br>Kaplan–Meier FFS rates:<br>3 y: 91%<br>5 y: 84%<br>8 y: 69%<br>PCa-specific survival: 100%<br>Overall survival: 100%<br>Metastasis-free survival: 99.6% | Not reported |

### 3.1. *Primary Intent*

In a first study [7], 16 patients with ages ranging from 40 to 78 were treated by using IRE. All patients were continent, and those who were potent before the operation remained potent after it. For two individuals who had bilateral regions treated, it took six months for their full potency to return. In 15 individuals (94%), postoperative biopsies from the site of confirmed malignancy revealed no sign of the disease.

After 12 months to IRE, all 16 of the males in the study by Valerio et al. [20] had pad-free and leak-free continence. The number of males who had an erection strong enough to penetrate dropped from 75% to 69%. There were no significant adverse effects noted. Changes in EPIC (Expanded Prostate Cancer Index Composite) and I-PSS (International Prostate Symptom Score) showed a statistically significant improvement in urine symptoms ($p = 0.039$ and 0.001, respectively).

Analogous results were obtained in another study [9], where 34 patients were recruited. A total of 100% (24/24) of patients were continent, and 95% (19/20) maintained their potency.

Between these patients, most of them had low or moderate risk disease (26% and 71%, respectively). A total of 6 months after the treatment, there were 12 Grade I (35%) and 10 Grade II (29%) complications. No patient experienced a problem of Grade III or more. The authors concluded by saying that additional prospective development studies are required to investigate the oncological potential and confirm the functional outcomes.

In order to indagate oncological outcomes, the study by Ting et al. [10] comprised 25 patients with low–intermediate-risk PCa who had not previously had PCa therapy. A total of 4% Grade III complications and 20% Grade 1 complications were discovered during follow-up. According to previous literature, no discernible change in American Urological Association urine symptom score, sexual function, or bowel function was seen at functional follow-up. No unusual abnormalities in-field in any of the patients were found after the treatment. No in-field recurrences occurred, and after 8 months, 76% of patients were histologically free of substantial malignancy. The treatment margins were widened to account for the fact that almost all recurrences occurred close to the treatment zone.

Collettini et al. [14] reported that there was no statistical difference in the proportion of men with preserved potency and leak-free and pad-free continence rates. According to modifications in the International Consultation on Incontinence Questionnaire Male Lower Urinary Tract Symptoms (ICIQ-MLUTS) and the International Index of Erectile Function (IIEF-5) questionnaires, urogenital function remained steady at 12 months. Multiparametric prostate MRI and targeted biopsies performed at 6 months revealed that the percentage of in-field treatment failure was 17.9%.

Being more specific about IRE complications, Murray et al. [11] reported 2 (8%) Grade III complications, including epididymitis and urinary tract infection, and 14 Grade II or lower complications (58%), including transitory urine symptoms, hematuria, and urinary tract infections. A total of 16% of the 25 patients developed malignancy in the ablation zone during regular follow-up biopsy at 6 months. Of those who had normal urine function at baseline, 88% and 94% reported having normal urinary function at 6 and 12 months following prostate gland ablation, respectively.

Van der Bos et al. [13] performed IRE ablation on high-volume disease with any Gleason sum score of 7 (ISUP Grades II–III) or any Gleason sum score of 6 (ISUP Grade I), including 63 patients in total. There were no high-grade adverse events according to the previous literature mentioned above. There was a little decline in the sexual QoL dimension (66 at baseline vs. 54 at 6 months, $p = 0.001$), but there was no significant change in the physical, mental, intestinal, or urinary QoL domains from baseline. On follow-up biopsies, the in-field and whole-gland oncological control rates were 84% (38/45 patients) and 76% (34/45 patients), respectively. They tried to find a reason for oncological failure of IRE ablation, and they reported that system faults ($p = 0.010$) and a small safety margin ($p = 0.047$) were shown to be possible early risk factors.

A recent study [16] valuated the IRE ablation of apical PCa lesions, including 50 patients who had a PCa lesion within 3 mm. In the EPIC urine or bowel QoL domain, there was no discernible difference between the baseline and 12-month post-treatment periods. A total of 12 months after therapy, one patient (2%) needed one pad per day to manage urine incontinence. EPIC sexual QoL decreased but not in a significantly way (from 65 at baseline to 59 at 12 months post-IRE). A total of 91% of the patients' pre-treatment potency persisted following therapy. Only one patient (2.5%) exhibited in-field residual disease.

Another study [15] analyzed 123 IRE-treated patients; of them, 76% exhibited no change in erectile function, and 98.8% continued to be pad-free. In-field recurrence was found in 2.7–9.8% of patients. Regarding FFS at three years, metastasis-free survival at that time was 99% and overall survival was 100%. A total of 18 patients required salvage therapy (12 underwent repeat IRE, and 6 underwent whole-gland therapy). Their conclusion was that focal IRE has acceptable short-term oncological results with little effect on patient quality of life in a subset of patients with localized clinically significant PCa.

A recent study [19] aimed to report both oncological and functional outcomes of IRE as the primary therapy for 223 locally advanced clinically significant PCa at a median follow-up of 5 years (up to 10 years). Short-term urine continence was maintained (98–99%); however, the number of erections strong enough for sexual activity fell by 13% from baseline (71% to 58%). Kaplan–Meier FFS rates were 91% at 3 years, 84% at 5 years, and 69% at 8 years. PCa-specific and overall survival were both 100%, whereas metastasis-free survival was 99.6%. Follow-up biopsy revealed residual PCa in 24% (45/190) of the cases. In this unique single-center longer-term follow-up, focused IRE showed acceptable local and distant oncological outcomes in a subset of males with less toxicity to the urinary system and sexual organs than radical therapy.

### 3.2. Salvage Intent after RT

In a single-center study [18], 74 males with biopsy-proven radio-recurrent PCa were treated with IRE. At the 12-month follow-up, 93% of the patients had maintained urine continence, and 23% had maintained erectile function. A total of 57 patients (77%) had local control and required no additional treatment. In-field recurrence occurred in 7% of patients, while out-field recurrence occurred in 15% of patients. A total of 91% of patients survived without developing metastases, with a median duration to metastases of 8 months. A sum of 60% was the predicted Kaplan–Meier 5-year progression-free survival rate. They came to the conclusion that these short- to mid-term safety, oncological, and quality-of-life outcome data support findings demonstrating the capacity of salvage-focused IRE to safely achieve oncological control in patients with radio-recurrent PCa.

### 3.3. Focal or Diffuse IRE?

In a study by de La Rosette et al. [17], in an investigation aimed at discerning the optimal approach for men with locally advanced, low-risk PCa, a meticulous randomization process was employed. This process led to the allocation of 51 patients to receive focused IRE ablation and 55 patients to undergo diffuse IRE. Quality-of-life assessments, utilizing measures such as IIEF-5, EPIC, and I-PSS, provided valuable insights into the comparative outcomes of these two distinct approaches.

Upon scrutinizing the data at the three-month follow-up, it was observed that rates of erectile dysfunction and adverse events were comparable between the two groups. Interestingly, the focal ablation group exhibited higher IIEF-5 scores, hinting at potential advantages in terms of erectile function within the initial three months. Notably, this observation was further supported by superior EPIC-sexual life scores in the focal ablation group compared to the extended ablation group.

However, it is crucial to highlight that other quality-of-life metrics did not show significant differences between the two groups, emphasizing the nuanced nature of the outcomes. The complexity of these results suggests that the impact of the ablation approach on various aspects of patients' lives is multifaceted and requires comprehensive evaluation.

A pivotal aspect of the study involved a 6-month prostate biopsy, a critical milestone in assessing the efficacy of the two ablation strategies. Surprisingly, no substantial differences were identified between the focal and prolonged IRE groups in terms of residual clinically relevant PCa (Gleason > 3 + 4), with rates standing at 18.8% and 13.2%, respectively.

In the conclusive remarks, the researchers asserted that among males with localized low–intermediate-risk PCa, both focal and diffuse IRE ablation exhibited comparable safety profiles, urinary function, and oncologic outcomes. The key differentiator emerged in the early phases of treatment, where focused ablation demonstrated superior outcomes in erectile function compared to diffuse ablation during the initial 3–6 months. These findings underscore the importance of considering not only long-term outcomes but also the early and nuanced impact of treatment choices on patients' quality of life.

## 4. Discussion

In order to prevent contractions during the IRE operation, a muscle relaxant agent is also administered to the patients under general anesthesia. A Foley catheter is placed to empty the bladder while the patient is in the lithotomy position, and it is maintained for at least two days following the treatment. The IRE console is composed by different monopolar needle electrodes and a direct current generator, and it is supervised by computer-based treatment planning software. Based on mpMRI and template-guided mapping prostate biopsies, preoperative targeted sites for ablation are identified [21].

The electrodes are positioned and guided in the predetermined targeted area using a trans-perineal template grid used for brachytherapy seed placement under ultrasound guidance. Following electrode insertion, IRE parameters, such as electrode exposure and distances between electrodes, are entered into the IRE system's planning software before IRE execution. The whole treatment takes around an hour.

To obtain a current flow of 20–50 A between each electrode pair, the IRE technique contain 90 pulses, each lasting 70 msec. The electrodes are carefully removed after the energy transfer, leaving the urine catheter in situ. Depending on the size of the ablation zone and its proximity to the intraprostatic urethra, the urine catheter is withdrawn 2–10 days following the treatment.

Collettini et al., in their study [14], performed a transrectal contrast-material-enhanced US of the prostate utilizing the MRI-transrectal/US-fusion method the day before and the day after IRE in order to evaluate the perfusion changes within the predefined target volume during all the procedure.

Neal et al. [8] administered prostate IRE protocols to two human malignant prostates and a healthy canine prostate while monitoring electrical data. With a treatment volume that demonstrates fast lesion development and resolution, there is a sub-millimeter boundary between damaged and unaffected cells that is tunable based on electrode configurations and pulse settings. Treatment planning is made by the correlation between the destroyed volume and the distribution of the electric field, and real-time treatment monitoring is made by alterations in tissue properties. The electroporated tissue may trigger a supplemental immunological response. Crucially, the extracellular matrix is unaffected by the pulses, protecting delicate anatomical regions such the ductal structures, neurovascular bundles, and main arteries. Because of this, locations that are too risky for resection or other focused procedures can be treated with IRE with a low risk of morbidity.

In tiny animals, IRE has showed its usefulness in treating complicated malignancies in delicate areas. These include a brain tumor and a sizable sarcoma that covered the sciatic nerve and important blood arteries. As looked at in the short- and medium-term, IRE safely ablated both malignant human prostates and healthy canine prostates. In the human cases, the histological results reveal instances of full tissue necrosis in the center with varying tissue damage outside the periphery.

Onik et al. [7] used IRE in sixteen individuals between the ages of 40 and 78. Every patient was treated as an outpatient and had good tolerance for the treatment. The treated area had variable echogenicity, according to US collected during the surgery. When the prostatic capsule was included in the formed lesion, it was seen to be indistinct. Immediately following the surgery, color Doppler ultrasonography revealed unbroken flow inside the neurovascular bundle. There was a range of 0 to 3 days in the catheter drainage period. The patient who underwent treatment for lesions on both sides of the gland experienced the greatest duration. After the treatment, every patient who was potent prior to it became potent again. All patients were continent immediately following treatment.

The biopsy specimens obtained after IRE whole-gland treatment showed no signs of any functional glandular tissue. There were occasionally parenchymal areas with the ghostly remains of glandular structures; however, there was no presence of living cells. Intact nerve bundles and living ganglion cells were observed, encircled by fibrotic and necrotic tissue. Vascular components were also present and unobstructed.

In their study, van den Bos et al. proposed radical prostatectomy as scheduled to take place four weeks after IRE on 16 individuals with PCa [13]. The macroscopic examination discerned a distinct ellipsoid-shaped hemorrhagic region enveloping petite pale discolored zones situated at the center of the IRE ablation zone. Notably, the ablation volumes, exhibiting well-defined demarcation, spanned a spectrum from 5 to 40% of the prostate, extending comprehensively from the capsule to the prostatic urethra. It is noteworthy that one prostate specimen did not manifest any macroscopically assessable ablation zone, and the tracts of the electrodes were indiscernible. Upon microscopic scrutiny of the ablation zone, it was elucidated that fibrosis, necrosis, and ghost-tubuli with eosinophilic cytoplasm were discernible in 15 out of 16 patients. This region was encapsulated by a hemorrhagic area, corresponding with the precise location of the electrodes as identified through ultrasound imaging. Importantly, the ablation zone exhibited a well-demarcated nature, featuring a sharply defined boundary that delineated the viable and non-viable tissue zones. A singular prostate specimen solely exhibited fibrosis without a necrotic component. Additionally, the ablated tissue showcased mild to moderate inflammation across all cases, with one case displaying a focal severe inflammatory component characterized by atrophic cells. Glandular hyperplasia was evident in 11 prostates, and further histological analysis identified basal cell hyperplasia and transitional cell metaplasia in 10 and 1 cases, respectively. Importantly, no skip lesions, indicative of the absence of viable tissue, were observed within the ablated area. Pertinently, the IRE treatment impacted the prostate capsule in 12 out of 16 cases, showcasing invasion by adipocytes and lipophages within the capsule structure. The boundary between viable and nonviable tissue in the ablation zone was sharply defined. Mild to severe inflammation and, in one instance, atrophic cells were seen in the ablated tissue. At the site of the electrodes, there was bleeding all around the region. Thirteen individuals had fibrinoid necrosis of the neurovascular bundle, and nine had denudation of the urothelium of the prostatic urethra.

In primary-intent IRE, the in-field recurrence is quite low (ranges from 0% to 33%). Urinary continence after the treatment remains high (>86%). Due to several different patients in the studies, the preserved potency varied by quite a lot (59–100%). Regarding complications, the highest are Grades I and II (20–77% and 0–29%, respectively). Grade III complications are less than 7%. About the specific oncological outcomes, both PCa-specific survival and overall survival is 100%. Metastasis-free survival is 99.6%. In a long-term study, the Kaplan–Meier FFS rates reported are 91% at 3 years, 84% at 5 years, and 69% at 8 years.

In the single study with salvage-intent IRE, the in-field recurrence was 7%. The urinary continence was still high (93%), but preserved potency was significantly lower than primary-intent IRE patients (23%). In addition, Grade III complications were slightly higher (10.8%).

Scheltema et al. [12] compared clinical outcomes of IRE patients vs. radical prostatectomy patients. In terms of maintaining pad-free continence and erections strong enough for intercourse, IRE was noticeably superior to radical prostatectomy. There were no statistically significant differences between the EPIC summary scores. Grade I complications were 22% and 16% for IRE and RP, respectively; Grade II complications were 13.7% and 9% for IRE and RP, respectively; there were no Grade III complications for either IRE or RP. Despite IRE patients initially complaining more, urinary symptoms for both groups of patients were improved after 12 months. A limitation is that individuals with IRE had more early oncological failure than individuals with radical prostatectomy.

In the comprehensive examination of treatments, a detailed comparative review [22] between Irreversible Electroporation (IRE) and High-Intensity Focused Ultrasound (HIFU) has unveiled intriguing insights into their respective outcomes. Patients undergoing IRE exhibited notable advantages, including higher mean rates of in-field negative post-treatment biopsy results, lower mean prostate-specific antigen (PSA) level decreases, and superior rates of potency maintenance compared to their HIFU counterparts. The nuanced analysis of adverse events further enriched the comparison. Commonly reported issues, such as urinary tract infection, dysuria, hematuria, and incontinence or urgency, were prevalent in both IRE and HIFU treatments. Remarkably, the majority of these adverse events were categorized as equivalent and mild, falling within Grades I or II. This underscores the overall safety profile of both treatments, emphasizing the manageable nature of the reported side effects. Delving deeper into the safety assessment, it is noteworthy that after IRE and HIFU procedures, only a modest percentage of patients, ranging from 0 to 8%, experienced serious adverse events categorized as Grade III. This low incidence of severe complications suggests a favorable risk profile for both IRE and HIFU, highlighting their suitability for individuals seeking minimally invasive treatment options for prostate-related conditions. Equally important, both IRE and HIFU demonstrated commendable functional results and showcased their ability to preserve the quality of life (QoL) for treated individuals. This positive outcome is crucial in the evaluation of treatment modalities, as it indicates not only the therapeutic efficacy but also the holistic impact on patients' well-being. As the scientific community continues to scrutinize the intricacies of IRE and HIFU, this comparative analysis serves as a valuable reference for clinicians and researchers alike. The ongoing pursuit of understanding the nuanced differences and similarities between these innovative treatment approaches will undoubtedly contribute to the refinement and optimization of prostate care, ultimately offering patients a spectrum of choices tailored to their individual needs and preferences.

## 5. Conclusions

In males diagnosed with localized low–intermediate-risk prostate cancer, IRE has demonstrated an exceptional safety profile and the potential for favorable outcomes in terms of both sexual and urinary function. The short-term oncological results of IRE are encouraging, suggesting its viability as a therapeutic option. Particularly noteworthy is the positive impact of IRE on patients with unifocal localized clinically significant PCa. This advanced technology may offer a pathway for these patients, allowing over 80% of them to sidestep more drastic therapeutic interventions even after a 5-year follow-up period. The appeal of IRE is evident, especially among individuals with screen-detected cancer who possess unifocal, favorable, low-volume, intermediate-risk disease. For many, IRE could potentially become the preferred initial course of treatment. Despite its promising prospects, widespread accessibility to IRE remains limited, currently confined to clinical trials and a select number of institutions. The potential benefits of this innovative treatment option are thus not yet available to the broader population. A future scenario where IRE is widely accessible could significantly alter the treatment landscape for men facing screen-detected cancer with specific disease characteristics. For the moment, the utilization of IRE hinges on more extensive multi-center trials and longer-term follow-up studies. These endeavors are crucial in establishing the broader effectiveness, safety, and sustained outcomes of IRE in the management of PCa. As this technology progresses through rigorous testing and evaluation, it holds the promise of becoming a mainstream and transformative therapeutic approach for a significant subset of PCa patients.

**Author Contributions:** Conceptualization, E.F. and D.S.; methodology, D.V.; software, D.V.; validation, E.F., D.S. and B.B.Z.; formal analysis, D.V.; investigation, F.V., E.V. and G.P.; resources, D.V.; data curation, D.V.; writing—original draft preparation, D.V.; writing—review and editing, D.S. and E.F.; visualization, D.V.; supervision, R.F.G. and B.B.Z.; project administration, E.F. All authors have read and agreed to the published version of the manuscript.

**Funding:** This research received no external funding.

**Institutional Review Board Statement:** Not applicable.

**Informed Consent Statement:** Not applicable.

**Data Availability Statement:** Data is contained within the article.

**Conflicts of Interest:** The authors declare no conflict of interest.

## Abbreviations

| | |
|---|---|
| EMBASE | Excerpta Medica dataBASE |
| EBRT | External beam radiation therapy |
| EPIC | Expanded Prostate Cancer Index Composite |
| HIFU | High-intensity focused ultrasound |
| ICIQ-MLUTS | International Consultation on Incontinence Questionnaire Male Lower Urinary Tract Symptoms |
| IIEF-5 | International Index of Erectile Function |
| I-PSS | International Prostate Symptom Score |
| IRE | Irreversible electroporation |
| ISUP | Internetional Society of Urologist pathologists |
| MEDLINE | Medical Literature Analysis and Retrieval System Online |
| mpMRI | Multiparametric magnetic resonance imaging |
| PCa | Prostate Cancer |
| QoL | Quality of life |
| RP | Radical prostatectomy |
| RT | Radiotherapy |
| TRUS | Trans-rectal ultrasound |

## References


1. Linares-Espinós, E.; Carneiro, A.; Martínez-Salamanca, J.I.; Bianco, F.; Castro-Alfaro, A.; Cathelineau, X.; Valerio, M.; Sanchez-Salas, R. New technologies and techniques for prostate cancer focal therapy. *Minerva Urol. Nephrol.* **2018**, *70*, 252–263. [CrossRef]
2. Lodeizen, O.; de Bruin, M.; Eggener, S.; Crouzet, S.; Ghai, S.; Varkarakis, I.; Katz, A.; Dominguez-Escrig, J.L.; Pahernik, S.; de Reijke, T.; et al. Ablation energies for focal treatment of prostate cancer. *World J. Urol.* **2019**, *37*, 409–418. [CrossRef] [PubMed]
3. Ahmed, H.U.; El-Shater Bosaily, A.; Brown, L.C.; Gabe, R.; Kaplan, R.; Parmar, M.K.; Collaco-Moraes, Y.; Ward, K.; Hindley, R.G.; Freeman, A.; et al. Diagnostic accuracy of multi-parametric MRI and TRUS biopsy in prostate cancer (PROMIS): A paired validating confirmatory study. *Lancet* **2017**, *389*, 815–822. [CrossRef] [PubMed]
4. Kasivisvanathan, V.; Rannikko, A.S.; Borghi, M.; Panebianco, V.; Mynderse, L.A.; Vaarala, M.H.; Briganti, A.; Budäus, L.; Hellawell, G.; Hindley, R.G.; et al. MRI-Targeted or Standard Biopsy for Prostate-Cancer Diagnosis. *N. Engl. J. Med.* **2018**, *378*, 1767–1777. [CrossRef] [PubMed]
5. Wagstaff, P.G.K.; de Bruin, D.M.; van den Bos, W.; Ingels, A.; van Gemert, M.J.C.; Zondervan, P.J.; Verdaasdonk, R.M.; van Lienden, K.P.; van Leeuwen, T.G.; de la Rosette, J.J.M.C.H.; et al. Irreversible electroporation of the porcine kidney: Temperature development and distribution. *Urol. Oncol. Semin. Orig. Investig.* **2015**, *33*, 168.e1–168.e7. [CrossRef] [PubMed]
6. Lee, E.W.; Thai, S.; Kee, S.T. Irreversible Electroporation: A Novel Image-Guided Cancer Therapy. *Gut Liver* **2010**, *4* (Suppl. S1), S99. [CrossRef] [PubMed]
7. Onik, G.; Rubinsky, B. Irreversible Electroporation: First Patient Experience Focal Therapy of Prostate Cancer. In *Irreversible Electroporation*; Series in Biomedical Engineering; Springer: Berlin/Heidelberg, Germany, 2010; pp. 235–247. [CrossRef]
8. Neal, R.E.; Millar, J.L.; Kavnoudias, H.; Royce, P.; Rosenfeldt, F.; Pham, A.; Smith, R.; Davalos, R.V.; Thomson, K.R. In vivo characterization and numerical simulation of prostate properties for non-thermal irreversible electroporation ablation. *Prostate* **2014**, *74*, 458–468. [CrossRef] [PubMed]
9. Valerio, M.; Stricker, P.D.; Ahmed, H.U.; Dickinson, L.; Ponsky, L.; Shnier, R.; Allen, C.; Emberton, M. Initial assessment of safety and clinical feasibility of irreversible electroporation in the focal treatment of prostate cancer. *Prostate Cancer Prostatic Dis.* **2014**, *17*, 343–347. [CrossRef]
10. Ting, F.; Tran, M.; Böhm, M.; Siriwardana, A.; Van Leeuwen, P.J.; Haynes, A.-M.; Delprado, W.; Shnier, R.; Stricker, P.D. Focal irreversible electroporation for prostate cancer: Functional outcomes and short-term oncological control. *Prostate Cancer Prostatic Dis.* **2016**, *19*, 46–52. [CrossRef]
11. Murray, K.S.; Ehdaie, B.; Musser, J.; Mashni, J.; Srimathveeravalli, G.; Durack, J.C.; Solomon, S.B.; Coleman, J.A. Pilot Study to Assess Safety and Clinical Outcomes of Irreversible Electroporation for Partial Gland Ablation in Men with Prostate Cancer. *J. Urol.* **2016**, *196*, 883–890. [CrossRef]
12. Scheltema, M.J.; Chang, J.I.; Böhm, M.; van den Bos, W.; Blazevski, A.; Gielchinsky, I.; Kalsbeek, A.M.F.; van Leeuwen, P.J.; Nguyen, T.V.; de Reijke, T.M.; et al. Pair-matched patient-reported quality of life and early oncological control following focal irreversible electroporation versus robot-assisted radical prostatectomy. *World J. Urol.* **2018**, *36*, 1383–1389. [CrossRef] [PubMed]
13. van den Bos, W.; Jurhill, R.R.; de Bruin, D.M.; Savci-Heijink, C.D.; Postema, A.W.; Wagstaff, P.G.K.; Muller, B.G.; Varkarakis, I.M.; Skolarikos, A.; Zondervan, P.J.; et al. Histopathological Outcomes after Irreversible Electroporation for Prostate Cancer: Results of an Ablate and Resect Study. *J. Urol.* **2016**, *196*, 552–559. [CrossRef]
14. Collettini, F.; Enders, J.; Stephan, C.; Fischer, T.; Baur, A.D.J.; Penzkofer, T.; Busch, J.; Hamm, B.; Gebauer, B. Image-guided Irreversible Electroporation of Localized Prostate Cancer: Functional and Oncologic Outcomes. *Radiology* **2019**, *292*, 250–257. [CrossRef]

15. Blazevski, A.; Scheltema, M.J.; Yuen, B.; Masand, N.; Nguyen, T.V.; Delprado, W.; Shnier, R.; Haynes, A.-M.; Cusick, T.; Thompson, J.; et al. Oncological and Quality-of-life Outcomes Following Focal Irreversible Electroporation as Primary Treatment for Localised Prostate Cancer: A Biopsy-monitored Prospective Cohort. *Eur. Urol. Oncol.* **2020**, *3*, 283–290. [CrossRef] [PubMed]
16. Blazevski, A.; Amin, A.; Scheltema, M.J.; Balakrishnan, A.; Haynes, A.-M.; Barreto, D.; Cusick, T.; Thompson, J.; Stricker, P.D. Focal ablation of apical prostate cancer lesions with irreversible electroporation (IRE). *World J. Urol.* **2021**, *39*, 1107–1114. [CrossRef] [PubMed]
17. de la Rosette, J.; Dominguez-Escrig, J.; Zhang, K.; Teoh, J.; Barret, E.; Ramon-Borja, J.C.; Muir, G.; Bohr, J.; de Reijke, T.; Ng, C.-F.; et al. A Multicenter, Randomized, Single-blind, 2-Arm Intervention Study Evaluating the Adverse Events and Quality of Life After Irreversible Electroporation for the Ablation of Localized Low-intermediate Risk Prostate Cancer. *J. Urol.* **2023**, *209*, 347–353. [CrossRef] [PubMed]
18. Geboers, B.; Scheltema, M.J.; Blazevski, A.; Katelaris, A.; Doan, P.; Ali, I.; Agrawal, S.; Barreto, D.; Matthews, J.; Haynes, A.; et al. Median 4-year outcomes of salvage irreversible electroporation for localized radio-recurrent prostate cancer. *BJU Int.* **2023**, *131*, 14–22. [CrossRef]
19. Scheltema, M.J.; Geboers, B.; Blazevski, A.; Doan, P.; Katelaris, A.; Agrawal, S.; Barreto, D.; Shnier, R.; Delprado, W.; Thompson, J.E.; et al. Median 5-year outcomes of primary focal irreversible electroporation for localised prostate cancer. *BJU Int.* **2023**, *131*, 6–13. [CrossRef]
20. Valerio, M.; Dickinson, L.; Ali, A.; Ramachadran, N.; Donaldson, I.; Mccartan, N.; Freeman, A.; Ahmed, H.U.; Emberton, M. Nanoknife Electroporation Ablation Trial: A Prospective Development Study Investigating Focal Irreversible Electroporation for Localized Prostate Cancer. *J. Urol.* **2017**, *197 (3 Part 1)*, 647–654. [CrossRef]
21. Edd, J.F.; Horowitz, L.; Davalos, R.V.; Mir, L.M.; Rubinsky, B. In Vivo Results of a New Focal Tissue Ablation Technique: Irreversible Electroporation. *IEEE Trans. Biomed. Eng.* **2006**, *53*, 1409–1415. [CrossRef]
22. Cribbs, K.A.; Manning, E.F.; Zhou, J.; Lahue, B.J.; Polascik, T.J. Real-World Comparative Safety and Effectiveness of Irreversible Electroporation and High-Intensity Focused Ultrasound for Prostate Cancer Ablation. *Urology* **2023**, *174*, 7–17. [CrossRef]

MDPI AG
Grosspeteranlage 5
4052 Basel
Switzerland
Tel.: +41 61 683 77 34

*Journal of Personalized Medicine* Editorial Office
E-mail: jpm@mdpi.com
www.mdpi.com/journal/jpm

www.ingramcontent.com/pod-product-compliance
Lightning Source LLC
Chambersburg PA
CBHW062103220926
51850CB00010B/2873
* 9 7 8 3 7 2 5 8 6 4 0 0 3 *